ETHICS IN PARTICIPATORY RESEARCH FOR HEALTH AND SOCIAL WELL-BEING

Participatory research is well-established as an approach involving people with a direct interest in, or experience of, the issue being studied in carrying out research. However, it raises unique and challenging ethical issues. Traditional concerns with respect for the rights to confidentiality, consent, privacy and protection of 'research informants' do not translate easily into participatory research. Boundaries between researchers and those researched are often blurred; research trajectories may be emergent and unpredictable; and major ethical issues revolve around partnership, power, equality and respect for diverse knowledges.

This book introduces the key ethical issues in participatory research, drawing on ethical theory and relevant literature before presenting seven substantive chapters, each on a different theme, such as power, ownership, confidentiality and boundaries. The chapters feature an introductory overview of the topic with reference to the literature, followed by four real-life case examples written by participatory researchers and short commentaries on each case. Drawn from around the world (from Denmark to Tanzania), the cases illustrate a range of ethical issues, outlining how they were handled and the reflections and feelings of the contributors.

Focusing on developing ethical awareness, confidence and courage to act in ethically challenging situations in everyday research practice, this book is an invaluable resource for all participatory researchers.

Sarah Banks is Professor of Applied Social Sciences, Department of Sociology and Co-director, Centre for Social Justice and Community Action, Durham University, UK.

Mary Brydon-Miller is Professor of Educational Leadership, Evaluation, and Organizational Development, College of Education and Human Development, University of Louisville, USA.

ETHICS IN PARTICIPATORY RESEARCH FOR HEALTH AND SOCIAL WELL-BEING

Cases and Commentaries

Edited by Sarah Banks and Mary Brydon-Miller

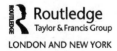

Routledge
Taylor & Francis Group

LONDON AND NEW YORK

First published 2019
by Routledge
2 Park Square, Milton Park, Abingdon, Oxon OX14 4RN

and by Routledge
711 Third Avenue, New York, NY 10017

Routledge is an imprint of the Taylor & Francis Group, an informa business

British Library Cataloguing-in-Publication Data
A catalogue record for this book is available from the British Library

Library of Congress Cataloging-in-Publication Data
Names: Banks, Sarah, editor. | Brydon-Miller, Mary, editor. Title: Ethics in participatory research for health and social well-being : cases and commentaries / edited by Sarah Banks and Mary Brydon-Miller. Description: Abingdon, Oxon ; New York, NY : Routledge, 2018. | Includes bibliographical references and index. Identifiers: LCCN 2018013419| ISBN 9781138093416 (hbk) | ISBN 9781138093430 (pbk) | ISBN 9781315106847 (ebk) Subjects: | MESH: Biomedical Research--ethics | Community-Based Participatory Research--ethics | Ethics, Research | Principle-Based Ethics | Human Rights | Case Reports Classification: LCC R724 | NLM W 20.55.E7 | DDC 174.2--dc23LC record available at https://lccn.loc.gov/2018013419

ISBN: 978-1-138-09341-6 (hbk)
ISBN: 978-1-138-09343-0 (pbk)
ISBN: 978-1-315-10684-7 (ebk)

Typeset in Bembo
by Servis Filmsetting Ltd, Stockport, Cheshire

TABLE OF CONTENTS

List of tables   xii
Notes on contributors   xiii
Preface and acknowledgements   xx

1 Ethics in participatory research   1
    Sarah Banks and Mary Brydon-Miller

2 Partnership, collaboration and power   31
    *Barbara Groot and Tineke Abma, with cases contributed by Annette
    Bilfeldt, Jackie Robinson, Jenevieve Mannell and Candice Satchwell,
    and additional commentaries by Melanie Peterman and Ruud van Zuijlen*

    Part 1 Introduction and overview of the issues   31
    Barbara Groot and Tineke Abma

    Part 2 Cases and commentaries   40

    Case 2.1 Power inequities and ethical challenges in action research at
    public nursing homes in Denmark, *Annette Bilfeldt*   40

    Commentary on Case 2.1, *Barbara Groot, Melanie Peterman, Ruud van
    Zuijlen and Tineke Abma*   42

Case 2.2 Participatory research with adults with Asperger's syndrome in the UK, *Jackie Robinson*   43

Commentary on Case 2.2, *Barbara Groot, Melanie Peterman, Ruud van Zuijlen and Tineke Abma*   45

Case 2.3 Researching gender-based violence in Rwanda: What do we really mean by 'building' local research capacity? *Jenevieve Mannell*   46

Commentary on Case 2.3, *Barbara Groot, Melanie Peterman, Ruud van Zuijlen and Tineke Abma*   48

Case 2.4 Starting as you mean to go on: Including young people in a participatory research project in the UK, *Candice Satchwell*   49

Commentary on Case 2.4, *Barbara Groot, Melanie Peterman, Ruud van Zuijlen and Tineke Abma*   51

Part 3 Concluding comments   **52**
Barbara Groot and Tineke Abma

3 Blurring the boundaries between researcher and researched, academic and activist   56
Anne MacFarlane and Brenda Roche, with cases contributed by Pinky Shabangu, Catherine Wilkinson, Mieke Cardol and Geralyn Hynes

Part 1 Introduction and overview of the issues   **56**
Anne MacFarlane and Brenda Roche

Part 2 Cases and commentaries   **64**

Case 3.1 Following research protocols versus being sensitive to informants' feelings: Ethical issues for a community researcher in Southern Africa, *Pinky Shabangu*   64

Commentary on Case 3.1, *Anne MacFarlane and Brenda Roche*   65

Case 3.2 Are you telling me this as a researcher or a friend? Ethical issues for a UK doctoral researcher, *Catherine Wilkinson*   66

Commentary on Case 3.2, *Anne MacFarlane and Brenda Roche*   68

Case 3.3 The power and dilemmas of 'in between' and off-the-
record: Participatory research with people with intellectual disabilities
in The Netherlands, *Mieke Cardol*   69

Commentary on Case 3.3, *Anne MacFarlane and Brenda Roche*   72

Case 3.4 When research becomes a therapeutic intervention: Using
PhotoVoice in an Irish hospital, *Geralyn Hynes*   73

Commentary on Case 3.4, *Anne MacFarlane and Brenda Roche*   75

Part 3 Concluding comments   **76**
Anne MacFarlane and Brenda Roche

4 Community rights, conflict and democratic representation   80
*Meghna Guhathakurta with cases contributed by Angela Contreras,
Shaun Cleaver, Michael J. Kral, Monika Bjeloncikova and Vendula
Gojova*

Part 1 Introduction and overview of the issues   **80**
Meghna Guhathakurta

Part 2 Cases and commentaries   **89**

Case 4.1 Doing research, advocating for human rights, and
preserving community relations amongst migrant workers in Canada:
A silence that (still) bothers, *Angela Contreras*   89

Commentary on Case 4.1, *Meghna Guhathakurta*   91

Case 4.2 Whose voice is included and whose should be loudest?
Negotiating value systems with respect to leadership and membership
in rural Zambia, *Shaun Cleaver*   92

Commentary on Case 4.2, *Meghna Guhathakurta*   94

Case 4.3 Suicide and well-being: A participatory study with Inuit in
Arctic Canada, *Michael J. Kral*   95

Commentary on Case 4.3, *Meghna Guhathakurta*   97

Case 4.4 Working with community conflict and ethnic tensions in a
'socially excluded locality' in the Czech Republic, *Monika Bjeloncikova
and Vendula Gojova*   97

Commentary on Case 4.4, *Meghna Guhathakurta*   97

Part 3 Concluding comments   **101**
Meghna Guhathakurta

5 Co-ownership, dissemination and impact   103
*Gustaaf Bos and Tineke Abma, with cases contributed by Kate York,
Sarah Marie Wiebe, Aila-Leena Matthies, Gustaaf Bos and Rafaella
van den Bosch, and additional commentaries by Truus Teunissen and
Doortje Kal*

Part 1 Introduction and overview of the issues   **103**
Gustaaf Bos and Tineke Abma

Part 2 Cases and commentaries   **112**

Case 5.1 Disagreements about ownership of data and use of findings:
Ethical issues in community-based health research in Tanzania, *Kate York* 112

Commentary on Case 5.1, *Tineke Abma, Truus Teunissen, Doortje Kal
and Gustaaf Bos*   115

Case 5.2 Decolonizing research through documentary film?
Indigenous environmental justice and community-engagement in
Canada, *Sarah Marie Wiebe*   116

Commentary on Case 5.2, *Tineke Abma, Truus Teunissen, Doortje Kal
and Gustaaf Bos*   119

Case 5.3 Two realities meeting one another: Young service users and
policy-makers in Finland, *Aila-Leena Matthies*   119

Commentary on Case 5.3, *Tineke Abma, Truus Teunissen, Doortje Kal
and Gustaaf Bos*   122

Case 5.4 About the 'co' in co-writing: Challenges for a Dutch
university researcher co-researching with people with intellectual
disabilities, *Gustaaf Bos and Rafaella van den Bosch*   122

Commentary on Case 5.4, *Tineke Abma, Truus Teunissen and Doortje Kal*   125

Part 3 Concluding comments   **125**
Tineke Abma and Gustaaf Bos

6 Anonymity, privacy and confidentiality   131
*Kristin Kalsem with cases contributed by Alana Martin, Christine
Lalonde, Lisa Boucher, Claire Kendall, Zack Marshall, Sarah
Switzer, Carol Strike, Adrian Guta, Soo Chan Carusone, Michelle
Brear, and Vu Song Ha*

Part 1 Introduction and overview of the issues   **131**
Kristin Kalsem

Part 2 Cases and commentaries   **139**

Case 6.1 Handling a privacy breach and participant notification:
Challenges for a community-based research project with people who
use drugs in Ottawa, Canada, *Alana Martin, Christine Lalonde, Lisa
Boucher, Claire Kendall, and Zack Marshall*   139

Commentary on Case 6.1, *Kristin Kalsem*   141

Case 6.2 Issues of confidentiality in working between research
and clinical care: Community-based research in an HIV hospital in
Toronto, Canada, *Sarah Switzer, Carol Strike, Adrian Guta, Soo Chan
Carusone*   143

Commentary on Case 6.2, *Kristin Kalsem*   145

Case 6.3 Tensions between confidentiality and equitable recognition
of co-researchers: Participatory health research in a Swazi village,
Michelle Brear   146

Commentary on Case 6.3, *Kristin Kalsem*   148

Case 6.4 Could we protect confidentiality, and for whom? Story
from a PhotoVoice project with teenagers living with Autism
Spectrum Disorder in Hanoi, Vietnam, *Vu Song Ha*   150

Commentary on Case 6.4, *Kristin Kalsem*   152

Part 3 Concluding comments   **153**
Kristin Kalsem

7 Institutional ethical review processes   155
Adrian Guta, with cases contributed by Colin Bradley, Anne
MacFarlane, Jane Jervis, Geralyn Hynes, and Jon Fieldhouse

Part 1 Introduction and overview of the issues   **155**
Adrian Guta

Part 2 Cases and commentaries   **165**

Case 7.1 Approving a participatory research proposal: Perspectives
from a Research Ethics Committee Chair and a researcher in Ireland,
Colin Bradley and Anne MacFarlane   165

Commentary on Case 7.1, *Adrian Guta*   167

Case 7.2 The question of parental consent for teenagers in a doctoral
research project in the UK, *Jane Jervis*   168

Commentary on Case 7.2, *Adrian Guta*   170

Case 7.3 Responding to concerns about participant burden and
vulnerability in health-related action research in Ireland, *Geralyn Hynes*   170

Commentary on Case 7.3, *Adrian Guta*   173

Case 7.4 Dilemmas in a UK PAR project involving mental health
service users and providers, *Jon Fieldhouse*   173

Commentary on Case 7.4, *Adrian Guta*   175

Part 3 Concluding comments   **176**
Adrian Guta

8 **Social action for social change**   181
   Erin Davis and Cathy Vaughan, with cases contributed by Saskia
   Duijs, Vivianne Baur, Raquel Ignacio, Philile Mbatha and Jasmin Chen

   Part 1 Introduction and overview of the issues   **181**
   Erin Davis and Cathy Vaughan

   Part 2 Cases and commentaries   **190**

   Case 8.1 Striving for social change through participatory research:
   Challenges in working in a multi-ethnic neighbourhood in The
   Netherlands, *Saskia Duijs and Vivianne Baur*   190

   Commentary on Case 8.1, *Erin Davis and Cathy Vaughan*   193

   Case 8.2 Shaking things up: Participatory research with women with
   disabilities in the Philippines, *Raquel Ignacio*   194

   Commentary on Case 8.2, *Erin Davis and Cathy Vaughan*   196

   Case 8.3 Research for social change: Developing understandings
   of conflicts between conservation and rural livelihoods in Kosi Bay,
   South Africa, *Philile Mbatha*   196

   Commentary on Case 8.3, *Erin Davis and Cathy Vaughan*   199

   Case 8.4 Researching community-led responses to family violence in
   Australia: Whose vision of socially just change? *Jasmin Chen*   200

   Commentary on Case 8.4, *Erin Davis and Cathy Vaughan*   202

   Part 3 Concluding comments   **203**
   Erin Davis and Cathy Vaughan

Index   207

LIST OF TABLES

Table 1.1   Some theoretical and methodological approaches to ethics   12
Table 1.2   Ethical principles for community-based participatory research   21
Table 1.3   Case-based exercises for use in learning and teaching   22

NOTES ON CONTRIBUTORS

Tineke Abma is Chair in 'Participation & Diversity' at VU University Medical Centre, Department of Medical Humanities and Amsterdam Public Health Institute, The Netherlands. Her work is grounded in responsive evaluation and care ethics. She has been involved in long-term projects in psychiatry (coercion reduction), elderly care (participation and empowerment) and chronic care and disability (patient autonomy and participation).

Sarah Banks is Professor of Applied Social Sciences, Department of Sociology and Co-director of the Centre for Social Justice and Community Action, Durham University, UK. She teaches and researches on ethics in social, community and youth work, and undertakes participatory action research in partnership with community organisations.

Vivianne Baur is Assistant Professor, Department of Care Ethics, University for Humanistic Studies in Utrecht, The Netherlands. Her research work in care institutions is based in a transformative research paradigm, using Participatory Action Research methodology to create dialogue, mutual understanding, and improve caring practices. She teaches academic writing and qualitative research methods.

Annette Bilfeldt is Associate Professor in Social Science and Social Innovation, Aalborg University in Copenhagen, Denmark. She is also affiliated with the Centre for Action Research and Democratic Social Change at Roskilde University, Denmark. Her research has focused on Participatory Action Research in public elder care. She is a member of the EU COST action ROSEnet Reducing Old Age Social Exclusion Network and the Danish Research Network at Aalborg University: The Centre for Democratic Ageing with Dignity.

Monika Bjelončíková is a PhD student in social work, Faculty of Social Studies, University of Ostrava. Her dissertation project focuses on life with HIV/AIDS and the challenges of the epidemic for social work. She is interested in participatory approaches in social work practically, theoretically and also in research.

Gustaaf Bos conducted PhD research on encounters between people with and without intellectual disabilities in 'reversed integration' settings. Since 2016 he has worked at the Department of Medical Humanities, VU University Medical Centre, Amsterdam, on participation and experiential knowledge of people with intellectual disabilities.

Lisa Boucher is a PhD student in Epidemiology and Public Health, University of Ottawa and Research Student at the Bruyère Research Institute. She completed her Master's in Cognitive Psychology at Carleton University and has worked with the PROUD research group since 2014. Her research interests include improving self-management support and equity in health and social service delivery for marginalised communities, in particular people living with, or at risk for, HIV.

Colin Bradley is Professor of General Practice (Family Medicine) in the School of Medicine, University College Cork, Ireland. In addition to clinical work in a small family practice he teaches a variety of health care students and carries out research. Main research interests are prescribing of medicines by primary health care professionals and primary care management of chronic diseases (particularly diabetes). He is former Chair of the Research Ethics Committee of the Irish College of General Practitioners and a member of several other ethics committees.

Michelle Brear is a postdoctoral research fellow, School of Education Studies, University of the Free State (Qwaqwa, South Africa) and Adjunct Research Fellow in the School of Public Health and Preventive Medicine, Monash University (Melbourne, Australia). Her research focuses on the process and outcomes of participatory research, particularly participation and empowerment.

Mary Brydon-Miller is Professor of Educational Leadership, Evaluation, and Organizational Development, College of Education and Human Development, University of Louisville, USA. Her current research focuses on engaging youth from around the world to act as citizen scientists to study the impacts of global climate change.

Mieke Cardol is Applied Science Professor of Disability Studies, Rotterdam University of Applied Sciences. She teaches and researches on experiential knowledge of people with a chronic condition, well-being and autonomy in the context of care and support, and diversity in societal participation. In the research she undertakes, people with a condition themselves often are co-researchers.

Soo Chan Carusone has a PhD in Health Research Methodology. She is Director of Research at Casey House and has a part-time appointment at McMaster University, Canada. As a mixed methods researcher based in a community-based HIV hospital she draws on academic–clinical–community partnerships in addressing issues of health equity and complex care in the context of HIV.

Jasmin Chen is Research Assistant at the Multicultural Centre for Women's Health, Melbourne, Australia. Her work includes community-based research and advocacy for immigrant and refugee women's health and well-being.

Shaun Cleaver is postdoctoral fellow in the School of Physical and Occupational Therapy, McGill University, Canada. His research focuses on disability, poverty, and policy, in collaboration with persons with disabilities in Western Zambia.

Angela M. Contreras is a community-based criminologist and evaluation practitioner and scholar. She is a doctoral fellow, Department of Educational Studies, University of British Columbia, Canada. Her current research concerns legislation, policies and conflicts around the provision of legal and digital literacy programmes and services for people with precarious migration and employment status in North and Central America.

Erin Davis is a Canadian–Australian social worker with a background in strategic policy advising, programme development and participatory research. Based in Melbourne, Australia, her work primarily involves addressing issues of gender equality and violence against women with a strong emphasis on feminist and social justice ethics.

Saskia Duijs is a junior researcher/PhD student at the Department of Medical Humanities, VU Medical Centre, Amsterdam. She has a Master's degree in Health Sciences and has conducted several participatory research projects on the recent transitions within the health and social care domain in the Netherlands.

Jon Fieldhouse is Senior Lecturer in Occupational Therapy, University of the West of England, Bristol, UK. His field of research is community-based mental health care and social inclusion for service users, and the use of participatory action research methodology.

Vendula Gojova is Assistant Professor, Department of Social Work, Faculty Social Studies, University of Ostrava, Czech Republic. She teaches and researches in ethnicity and diversity in social work. She contributes to participatory action research on so-called 'socially excluded localities'.

Barbara Groot is a researcher at VU University Medical Centre, Department of Medical Humanities and Amsterdam Public Health Institute, The Netherlands. She is working on her PhD thesis on Participatory Health Research and Ethics. Barbara coordinates the Centre of Client Experiences in Amsterdam and is involved in many participatory research projects in all different sectors. She teaches participatory and qualitative research.

Meghna Guhathakurta taught International Relations at the University of Dhaka, Bangladesh from 1984 to 2006. She is currently Executive Director of Research Initiatives, Bangladesh (RIB) a research support organisation based in Dhaka, which specialises in action research with marginalised and minority communities. She specialises in international development, gender relations and South Asian politics.

Adrian Guta is Assistant Professor, School of Social Work, University of Windsor, Canada. He regularly partners with clinical and community stakeholders to conduct research on the health care and social service needs of people living with HIV and people who use drugs. Adrian has written about ethical and methodological issues in community-engaged research.

Vu Song Ha is a medical doctor, public health specialist, and founder of the Center for Creative Initiatives in Health and Population (CCIHP), an NGO in Vietnam. She has implemented several participatory action research projects including visual art-based work with teenagers living with Autism Spectrum Disorder.

Geralyn Hynes is Associate Professor in Palliative Care and Director of Research, School of Nursing and Midwifery, Trinity College Dublin, Ireland. Her research interests are in action research and palliative care.

Raquel Ignacio is a Filipina researcher and activist, engaged in the Women's Movement in the Philippines for many years. A feminist, and passionate about social justice, she has worked in response to the trafficking of women, the exploitation of migrant workers, violence against women and the health and social inequalities experienced by communities living in informal settlements.

Jane Jervis is Lecturer in Nursing, Keele University, UK. Her current doctoral research involves using a participatory action research approach to improve the support provided to children and young people visiting adult relatives in hospital.

Doortje Kal was prevention worker, Social Psychiatry, 1992–2002. Her PhD was on welcoming people with a 'psychiatric background' [Kwartiermaken] in 2001. She was lector of 'Kwartiermaken' at the Utrecht University of Applied Sciences, 2011–2013. She is a member of the secretariat of the Dutch Researchers Platform 'Disability Studies, Inclusion & Belonging'. See http://www.kwartiermaken.nl/english for further information.

Kristin Kalsem is Charles Hartsock Professor of Law and Co-Director of the Center for Race, Gender, and Social Justice, University of Cincinnati College of Law, USA. She is currently working on two 'legal' participatory action research projects, one relating to predatory lending practices and the other to judicial training on domestic violence.

Claire Kendall is Associate Professor, Department of Family Medicine, University of Ottawa; Clinician Investigator, C.T. Lamont Primary Health Care Research Centre, Bruyère Research Institute and a practising family physician with the Bruyère Family Health Team. Her research aims to improve delivery of primary health care for populations with or at risk for HIV.

Michael Kral is Associate Professor, School of Social Work, Wayne State University, and on the faculty of the Department of Psychiatry, University of Toronto. He has conducted community-based participatory action research with Inuit in Arctic Canada for over 20 years.

Christine Lalonde has combined lived/work experience in marginalised communities and harm reduction. She has worked with the PROUD research team and various community health centres and service providers in Ottawa since 2014. Her special interests include peer engagement, research and advocacy.

Anne MacFarlane is Professor of Primary Healthcare Research in the Graduate Entry Medical School, University of Limerick, Ireland. She has expertise in participatory health research with socially excluded communities with a particular interest in migrants' involvement in health research.

Jenevieve Mannell is Lecturer in Global Health, University College London, UK. Her current research focuses on using participatory approaches to engage marginalised communities in gender-based violence prevention in low and middle income countries. She has active research projects in Peru, Afghanistan and Rwanda.

Zack Marshall is Assistant Professor, School of Social Work, McGill University, Canada. His work focuses on research ethics and participatory research, with particular attention to HIV, harm reduction, and the health of sexual and gender diverse individuals and communities.

Alana Martin combines lived/work experience in marginalised communities and harm reduction. She is research coordinator and cultural translator with the PROUD research group, of which she was a founding member. She has worked with community health centres and service providers since 2011 and is currently advocating for more meaningful peer engagement throughout Ottawa.

Aila-Leena Matthies is Professor of Social Work at the University of Jyväskylä, Kokkola University Consortium, Finland. She leads a qualifying MA and doctoral programme in Social Work. Research focuses on participatory approaches in welfare services and the ecosocial (environmental) perspective of social work. She is involved in a national practice project of participatory social work in Finland.

Philile Mbatha is Lecturer in the Environmental and Geographical Science Department, University of Cape Town, South Africa. She teaches and researches on rural development, rural livelihoods and natural ressource use in coastal environments, focusing on southern Africa.

Melanie Peterman has been co-researcher at the Centre of Client Experiences in Amsterdam, The Netherlands for three years. Melanie worked in the commercial sector until diagnosed with spinal cord injury in 2002. She has worked as a patient expert for 10 years, and also works as a life coach.

Brenda Roche is Director of Research at the Wellesley Institute, a Toronto-based think tank focused on advancing health equity through action on the social determinants of health. Brenda has expertise in medical anthropology and public health. Her research includes community-based and participatory research on health and social issues for urban populations, and currently focuses on health and working conditions for precarious workers.

Jackie Robinson is Principal Lecturer in Social Work, De Montfort University, Leicester, UK. Her research interests concern participatory research and research with people with Autism. Jackie also facilitates the Asperger's Consultation Group.

Candice Satchwell is Reader in Education and Literacies, University of Central Lancashire, UK. Current research is with disadvantaged young people to collect and tell stories about their lives.

Pinky N. Shabangu is a community-based researcher in Southern Africa. Research interests include innovative HIV prevention interventions for young women and girls. She is a Special Needs Teacher who holds a Diploma in Early Childhood Care and education and is completing a Bachelor of Education at the University of Swaziland.

Carol Strike, PhD, is Professor at the Dalla Lana School of Public Health, University of Toronto, and Affiliate Scientist, Centre for Urban Health Solutions, St. Michael's Hospital. Her research aims to improve health services for people who use drugs and other marginalised populations.

Sarah Switzer is a PhD candidate at the Faculty of Environmental Studies, York University, Canada. Her work focuses on arts-based and creative methods for engaging communities in research or community-based HIV or Harm Reduction programming. More broadly, her work touches on critical theory; participatory visual methods and ethics; and popular education.

Truus Teunissen is researcher at VU University Medical Centre, Department of Medical Humanities, Amsterdam. She combines her own experiential and scientific knowledge, focusing on perspectives of people with chronic illness or disability. She is involved in projects about health policy, societal relevance of research proposals, vulnerability, experiential knowledge and lived body experiences of people with chronic illnesses.

Rafaella van den Bosch is a 30-year-old woman with considerable life experience. As a trained assistant-researcher, she works for the Ben Sajet Centre in Amsterdam. Along with a researcher from the University of Amsterdam, she currently works with people with longstanding financial problems to gain insight into their life world and support needs.

Ruud van Zuijlen has lived with Multiple Sclerosis (MS) since he was a student. After finishing studies in Psychology, he facilitated self-help groups of MS patients. He was active in building the patient movement in Amsterdam, The Netherlands. After 30 years of experience as a patient expert, he is now a co-researcher at the Centre of Client Experiences in Amsterdam.

Cathy Vaughan is Senior Lecturer in Gender and Women's Health, Melbourne School of Population and Global Health, University of Melbourne, Australia. Her research and teaching focus on working with women in diverse settings to understand relationships between social contexts, gender relations and health.

Sarah Marie Wiebe grew up on Coast Salish territory in British Columbia, Canada. She is currently Assistant Professor, Department of Political Science, University of Hawai'i, Mānoa, where she focuses on environmental sustainability. Her book *Everyday Exposure: Indigenous Mobilization and Environmental Justice in Canada's Chemical Valley* (2016) won the Charles Taylor Book Award (2017).

Catherine Wilkinson is Lecturer in Children, Young People and Families, Faculty of Health and Social Care, Edge Hill University, UK. She is currently undertaking research with children and young people, around themes of health, identity, agency and participation.

Kate York is Assistant Professor of Clinical Nursing, University of Cincinnati College of Nursing and Director of Global Health Nursing. Kate returned to Tanzania to teach nursing at the Hubert Kairuki Memorial University in Dar es Salaam during 2014–2015.

PREFACE AND ACKNOWLEDGEMENTS

This book is the product of a complex and many-layered set of collaborations that have built from the bottom up. In this sense it mirrors the process of participatory research (PR), which is messy, unpredictable, emergent, and draws on and values many different types of knowledge and experience. As editors, it has been a privilege to work with the many committed and reflective participatory researchers from around the world who have contributed to the book. In the process of editing, our understandings of the micro-ethics of everyday PR practice have been immeasurably enhanced and our own levels of ethical awareness raised. We recommend the book to potential readers as a vehicle for enhancing ethical sensitivity, developing capacities for ethical reasoning, cultivating moral emotions, and improving the quality of PR processes.

Origins of the book

The stimulus for this book emerged from two research projects on ethics in community-based participatory research undertaken by the Centre for Social Justice and Community Action at Durham University, UK, in partnership with several other UK universities and community-based organisations during 2011–2012. Outputs included a literature review, ethical guidelines and a collection of UK ethics cases and commentaries.

While undertaking workshops and training sessions in the UK and around the world, case examples were particularly useful for stimulating ethical reflection and dialogue. Hence the Centre for Social Justice and Community Action began to collect longer, real-life cases relating to ethical challenges and dilemmas experienced by people engaging in participatory research. The idea of collecting cases was also taken up by the International Collaboration on Participatory Health Research (ICPHR), in which context the book project was conceived by Sarah Banks and developed over several annual working meetings of ICPHR during 2013–2017. Mary Brydon-Miller came on board as co-editor in 2015, having spent a term at Durham University as a visiting research fellow and bringing considerable expertise in the field of ethics in action research.

Who are we and what is our interest in ethics in PR?

Sarah Banks

I am a white woman with a background in community development and social work in the UK. My route into PR came from the practice of community development work, which involved working with groups of people gathering evidence to support challenges to existing social and political structures and initiate new developments. Sometimes this was called 'community research', but very often it was simply seen as an integral part of the community development and organising process. On joining Durham University, UK, initially as a Tutor in Community and Youth Work, I coordinated several research projects involving elements of youth peer research and later became involved in community-based participatory research (for example, working with community-based organisations researching and campaigning on household debt and poverty, facilitating co-inquiry groups on ethics in community-based participatory research, and co-producing research on historical and current aspects of civic engagement and community development). In 2009, several colleagues and I set up the Centre for Social Justice and Community Action at Durham University to support and promote participatory action research for social justice ends. My interest in practical ethics springs from a commitment to the value-based professional practice of community, youth and social work, combined with undergraduate studies in moral philosophy and experience in political campaigning and community organising. Having worked on professional ethics in social, community and youth work for several decades, I turned my attention to the ethical aspects of PR, taking the opportunity to apply with collaborators for small grants offered by the 'Connected Communities' programme of Research Councils UK, launched in 2010.

I was delighted to meet Mary Brydon-Miller when she attended our conference on ethics in community-based participatory research in Durham in 2013. As one of the few people writing creatively and seriously about ethics in action research, it was an exciting moment for me and my colleagues at CSJCA. Since then she has visited Durham on three further occasions, offering great support and inspiration to members of CSJCA and contributing very popular workshops, seminars and tutoring on our annual PAR course for doctoral researchers. Working with Mary as co-editor has broadened the scope of the book, bringing a wealth of experience and commitment to the complex task of editing.

Mary Brydon-Miller

Although I was unaware of it at the time, my first forays into participatory research began when I was an undergraduate student at the University of California, Santa Cruz studying the transportation needs of older residents of the city. Now the age of some of the people I spoke with then, I am still passionate about working to address pressing social, economic, and environmental issues here in my own home in Kentucky and around the world. My interest in research ethics grew out of my growing disillusionment with the formal research ethics processes in place within the university which fail to engage the very real ethical challenges of community-based research while imposing levels of regulation and oversight that simply amplify the power and privilege of the academy. And at the same time I was and remain wary of colleagues conducting community-based research who too often seem to believe that their intention to do good is all that is required of them in terms of ethical oversight. And so I come to be working on this volume with my dear friend Sarah Banks out of a sense of commitment to engaging deeply with the questions raised by the authors and contributors to this volume.

Acknowledgements

This book started with the collection of ethics cases, and these are the focal points of the book. We are extremely grateful to the authors of the cases for being willing to share such honest and reflective accounts. It is not easy to write about aspects of relationships that were problematic, including harms caused and mistakes made, alongside accounts of learning gained, and attempts to rectify ethical infringements and engage in respectful, responsible and critical practice. Each case went through several iterations and we would like to thank the authors for their patience and willingness to engage with the editors. We would also like to thank the authors of the chapter introductions and commentaries, who have so ably carried out the demanding brief of writing a thematic overview for each chapter and commenting on four cases. Their overviews of the key issues relating to their chapters and the many insights they offer are vital in placing the cases in context.

Sarah Banks

I am very grateful to the Arts and Humanities Research Council (UK) for funding two projects under the Connected Communities research programme: *CBPR: ethics and outcomes* (AH/J501057/1) and *Tackling ethical issues in CBPR* (AH/J006645/1) and to the collaborators who worked on those projects. I would particularly like to thank colleagues in the Centre for Social Justice and Community Action at Durham University, the *Imagine – connecting communities through research* project, Thrive Teesside, National Coordinating Centre for Public Engagement, UK Participatory Research Network and International Collaboration on Participatory Health Research for the many inspiring and supportive conversations, and participation in countless workshops and conferences which stimulated ethical thinking. I would also like to acknowledge the learning from participating in three biennial gatherings in Canada of the Community-College-University Expo (C2U Expo), which proved a fruitful ground for ethical conversations, new inspirations and collecting some cases. Numerous people from these networks and others have contributed to the thinking that lies behind this book, only a few of whom can be named: Andrea Armstrong, Shauna Butterworth, Kathleen Carter, Tina Cook, Heather Davidson, Sophie Duncan, Helen Graham, Budd Hall, Angie Hart, Claire Holmes, Amelia Lee, Paul Manners, Ann McNulty, Niamh Moore, Andrew Orton, Rachel Pain, Kate Pahl, Frances Rifkin, Andrew Russell, Jane Springett, Cheryl Stewart, Paul Ward, Will Wilson and Michael Wright.

Mary Brydon-Miller

I would like to acknowledge the Institute of Advanced Study, Durham University, UK, for the award of a Co-Fund Research Fellowship during April–June 2015. This gave me the opportunity to get to know Sarah and to become involved in the work of the Centre for Social Justice and Community Action. I would also like to thank the Fulbright Foundation and Keele University for giving me the opportunity to develop my scholarship in the area of ethics and action research and Bristol University for granting me a Benjamin Meaker Fellowship that allowed me to further this work. And finally, I'm grateful to so many colleagues, friends, and students who have challenged, questioned, supported, and cared for me along the way.

Sarah Banks, Durham, UK
Mary Brydon-Miller, Louisville, USA
31 January 2018

1

ETHICS IN PARTICIPATORY RESEARCH

Sarah Banks and Mary Brydon-Miller

Introduction

This chapter introduces the topic of ethics in participatory research (PR), providing a rationale for the book and an overview of each chapter. PR involves people whose lives are the subject of study in some or all aspects of research design, process, dissemination and impact, with a focus on generating socially just change. As such, it raises distinctive ethical issues linked with collaboration; sharing power; co-ownership of data, findings and impact; attribution of authorship; changing roles and relationships; handling institutional ethical review processes; and collective organising for change. In this chapter we elaborate briefly on these issues, discussing a range of different approaches to conceptualising and practising ethics in PR.

We argue that an approach to ethics that takes account of the character traits, motives and relationships of the people involved, and the particularities of the situations in which they are acting, provides a helpful framework for PR. This contrasts with abstract and principle-based approaches to ethics in research, as well as those that are regulatory and compliance-based. We explore character- and relationship-based approaches to ethics, including the ethics of care, virtue ethics, communitarian and covenantal ethics and their contribution to an 'everyday ethics' for PR. We discuss the nature of the 28 cases from real-life research practice that feature in the book, which are used to illustrate day-to-day ethical challenges faced by participatory researchers working in the fields of health and social well-being.

The book focuses on health and social well-being, as it was developed as a project of the International Collaboration for Participatory Health Research (ICPHR). However, 'health and social well-being' is broadly conceived, encompassing research involving medical interventions to more overtly radical social justice projects, which give voice to people experiencing oppression and taking action for change. Much PR, even if not carried out by people who self-identify as health or social researchers, has an impact on the health and social well-being of those who participate. Hence the book is also relevant to research that may be identified as educational participatory research, citizen science or organisational action research, for example, although we do not include examples from all these fields. It is a companion book to *Participatory Research for Health and Social Well-being* (Abma et al., 2019), which was co-authored by members of ICPHR and designed as an introductory text.

Rationale for the book

While PR is well-established as an approach that involves people with a direct interest in, or experience of, the issues being studied in carrying out some aspects of the research, it has until recently been a minority interest. It is now growing in popularity worldwide, particularly in the university sector, with academics and students increasingly researching in partnership with civil society organisations, often with a view to stimulating social change or 'impact' (changes in thinking, policy or practices attributable to the research).

However, the complexities of PR are often not fully appreciated, nor are the unique and challenging ethical issues it raises. Traditional concerns in research ethics about respect for rights to confidentiality, consent, privacy and protection of research 'subjects' or informants do not translate easily into PR, where boundaries between researcher and researched may be unclear, the research trajectory may be emergent and unpredictable, and major ethical issues revolve around partnership, power, equality and respect for diverse knowledges. Hence our aim in this book is to delve more deeply into the complex ethical issues that arise in the everyday practice of PR, with a view to stimulating readers' ethical awareness, and improving their capacities for ethical reflection and dialogue.

The book was conceived as a curated collection of ethics cases. The inclusion of real-life cases from participatory researchers is designed to ground consideration of ethical issues in the contexts in which they arise. This enables us to take account of the hopes, anxieties and dilemmas experienced by those involved, as well as decisions made, actions taken and post-hoc ethical evaluations of participants and readers. However, the 28 cases do not necessarily speak for themselves, nor do they encompass the full range of ethical issues that might arise in PR. Hence there are substantive introductions to each chapter, offering an overview of one or more broad themes, before four cases are presented, written by different authors from a range of countries and contexts. Each case is followed by a reflective commentary and the chapter then closes with some final remarks regarding the issues raised throughout the chapter.

Before summarising the content of the book at the end of this chapter, we first discuss the history and nature of PR and outline the conception we are using in this book. We then discuss briefly our understanding of 'ethics' and the history and nature of concerns about ethics in research, before considering the distinctive ethical issues arising in PR and what kinds of theoretical and practical approaches to ethics may be useful in this context.

Participatory research

Participatory research is a collaborative effort in which people whose lives are affected by the issues being researched are partners in designing, undertaking and disseminating research to influence socially just change. The process aims to be democratic, participatory, empowering and educational. There are many variations, with different names and histories. Here we offer a very brief and partial overview of some of the varieties and their origins.

PR is often categorised as a form of action research, which can be characterised as a family of collaborative research methodologies focused on achieving positive change in communities and organisations (Reason & Bradbury, 2008). Its origins lie in a number of different social movements and practices concerned with liberatory and anti-colonial struggles, popular education and literacy, community development, and organisational change. Although the term 'participatory research' only came into common use from the mid-1970s, community-based participatory research practices were developing in the 1960s and early 1970s (organisation-based action research much earlier). One of the most notable and radical strands is associated with Orlando Fals Borda (1925–2008, political activist and sociologist at National University of Bogotá), who undertook what he called 'action research', working for social and economic change alongside people living in 'peasant' communities in Colombia. He is credited with popularising the term 'participatory action research' in the late 1970s (for details of his work, see Fals Borda, 1987, 1988, 2001; Fals Borda & Rahman, 1991). However, by then the term 'participatory research' was already in use, the orgins of which Budd Hall (2005) traces to Tanzania, linking to the work of Marja-Liisa Swantz, with whom he worked when undertaking community development and adult education at the University of Dar es Salaam in the early 1970s. Swantz (1974) wrote a paper about 'participant research' with women, while the following year Hall (1975) used the term 'participatory research' as 'a descriptive term for a collection of varied approaches which shared a participatory ethos' in a paper published in a special issue of the magazine *Convergence* (Hall, 2005, p. 7). The International Participatory Research Network was founded in 1976 by Hall and others, gaining inspiration and momentum from the first conference on action research held in Cartagena (Colombia) in 1977, organised by Fals Borda (Hall & Tandon, 2018). Global links began to develop from this point, linking the practice and thinking of many different movements around the world, from the work of Paulo Freire in Brazil to Rajesh Tandon in India (Freire, 1972; Tandon, 2005).

Given the 'participatory turn' beginning in the 1970s and growing rapidly in the 1990s in the fields of development work, popular education and liberatory movements, the time was ripe for adopting participatory approaches to research, which gained momentum as networks developed. Early accounts of PR in North

America were published in the volume *Voices of Change: Participatory Research in the United States and Canada* (Park et al.,1993). This included descriptions of projects being carried out at the Highlander Research and Education Center in Tennessee focused on using participatory methods and adult education to address problems in the Appalachian region of the American South (Gaventa, 1993; Horton, 1993; Merrifield, 1993) and a discussion of feminist participatory research by Patricia Maguire (1987). Alongside feminist PR, there was also a growing awareness of the potential of PR in Indigenous communities in the global North, including Australia and New Zealand (e.g. Smith, 1999), and the need for a high degree of critical awareness and humility amongst non-Indigenous researchers working with First Nations people, as exemplified in Cases 4.3 and 5.2 in this book about work with the Inuit and Aamjiwnaang in Canada.

Already this brief account of the origins of PR demonstrates how different terms are used for similar practices, depending upon the traditions and contexts in which they developed. PR has always had a close relationship with community development and activism, often practised in international development contexts where particular approaches have developed, including participatory rural appraisal (PRA, later Participatory Reflection and Action), linked with the influential work of Robert Chambers (1994), and participatory learning and action (PLA). The term 'community-based research' (CBR) is used widely in North America, particularly Canada, while 'community-based participatory research' (CBPR) has come to be used largely in North America to refer to participatory health research (Coughlin et al., 2017; Wallerstein et al., 2017). In the UK, Banks et al. (2013) use the term CBPR more literally to encompass any type of research (not just health-related research) that is based in communities of place, identity or interest and engages community members as co-researchers in some way. The International Collaboration for Participatory Health Research (ICPHR, founded in 2009) uses the term 'participatory health research' rather than CBPR (International Collaboration for Participatory Health Research [ICPHR], 2013).

Our conception of PR is of research that is community-based (its rationale and key stakeholders lie in communities of place, interest or identity rather than in large institutions such as universities or hospitals) and value-based (it enacts principles of mutual respect, collaboration, equality and social justice, for example). We draw on Durham University's Centre for Social Justice and Community Action (CSJCA) ethical principles for CBPR, reproduced later in this chapter in Table 1.2, using the term 'CBPR' literally to mean PR that is community based (Centre for Social Justice and Community Action & National Coordinating Centre for Public Engagement, 2012). We also draw on ICPHR's first position paper outlining key characteristics of 'participatory health research', which are applicable to all PR, including that it is locally situated, collectively owned, and promotes critical reflexivity (ICPHR, 2013).

However, despite the fine rhetoric of social justice in academic texts and practice manifestos, it is important to stress that the extent to which PR adopts genuine power-sharing models or seeks to challenge radically the structures that embed poverty and inequality in societies varies enormously. It can be used as a tool to reach and control marginalised people and communities as much as for the 'powering of knowledge from the margins' to transform their lives and livelihoods (Thomas and Nararayan, 2015, p. 3). The current popularity of community–university research partnerships, which in some areas are becoming relatively 'mainstream' and institutionalised, brings with it the benefits of opening up universities and promoting 'knowledge democracy', alongside the dangers of co-option and control (Bivens, Haffenden and Hall, 2015).

The role of 'the community' in participatory research

Since 'community' is a focus of attention in PR, and is also a contested concept, we will say a few words here about 'community', whilst also drawing readers' attention to Chapter 4 of this book, which critically explores community rights, conflict and democratic representation. While there are numerous characterisations of 'community', a useful generic description is: 'collectivities of people with some but not necessarily all characteristics in common' (Banks et al., 2019). While 'community' has connotations of homogeneity and closeness, the idea that the collectivity may share only certain characteristics in common allows for elements of heterogeneity and diversity. Communities may comprise people living in the same geographical area (e.g. an urban neighbourhood, or a village), people with common interests (e.g. a hockey team, birdwatchers) or identities (e.g. Hindu religion, or lesbian women). 'Community' falls into the category of what Plant describes as an 'essentially contested concept' (Plant, 1974), with multiple descriptive meanings as listed above and an evaluative meaning, generally with positive connotations linked to care and cohesion (Banks & Butcher, 2013; Crow & Allan, 1994; Somerville, 2016). While this makes it a problematic concept, it continues to be deployed in everyday life and public policy to promote social inclusion and stress commonality. Yet the sense of identity and being cared about that is felt by members of communities can also amount to pressure to conform, and relies on members differentiating themselves from others outside their communities. In addition to solidarity with each other, members of communities also need to practise tolerance of non-members, seeing themselves as part of broader society in order to combat stigma, marginalisation, and violence based on characteristics such as ethnicity, religion, gender, sexuality, class, age or ability (Banks et al. 2019). These issues of inter- and intra-community conflict and tensions between individual and community rights, needs and interests are discussed and exemplified in Chapter 4.

As the cases in Chapter 4 demonstrate, communities take many forms and the types and levels of participation involved in PR must be designed to respond to these differences. While most examples in this book involve academic or other 'professional' researchers working in partnership with people in communities, PR is often undertaken by members of community organisations themselves, without outside partners. In other cases, communities or organisations already well-established before a research partnership begins may seek an outside researcher themselves to provide support, as was the case in Michael Kral's work described in Case 4.3 with the Inuit in Canada. In such cases, the role of the outside researcher may be grounded in skills development and data generation and analysis. In other situations, a particular issue or concern may be known to members of the community, but without an attempt to organise around it having been undertaken. In such instances a professional researcher coming into a group must first serve as community development worker or organiser in order to bring people together around a particular concern, as exemplified in Case 8.1 about isolated women of minority ethnic origins in a Dutch city. In still others, members of the community may be divided or in conflict regarding an issue, in which case the outside researcher's role may focus on mediation and conflict resolution, as in Case 4.4 about work with Roma people in the Czech Republic. Each of these roles requires a specific set of skills and each situation raises particular ethical challenges.. The roles may also change over time and people may find themselves taking on several, sometimes conflicting, roles (see Chapter 3 of this volume on blurring boundaries).

The cases in this book exemplify the many forms 'community participation' may take, from communities in control to community members engaging in participatory exercises designed by outside researchers. As discussed in Chapter 2 of this volume (on partnership, collaboration and power), in designing and undertaking PR, it is important that those involved give consideration to the types of research they wish to do and how different parties will work together. In a scoping study of CBPR, Durham Community Research Team (2011, p. 6) identified four points on a continuum of community participation in research:

1. Community-controlled and -managed research, no professional researchers involved.
2. Community-controlled research with professional researchers managed by and working for the community.
3. Co-production – equal partnership between professional researchers and community members.
4. Controlled by professional researchers but with greater or lesser degrees of community partnership, e.g.
   • Advisory group involved in design, dissemination.
   • Trained community researchers undertake some/all of data gathering, analysis, writing.
   • Professional researcher uses participatory methods (e.g. young people take photos).

In assessing the accounts of research in the literature reviewed for the scoping study (mainly in academic journals), the majority appeared to fall into the fourth category (controlled by professional researchers, with some degree of community participation) (Durham Community Research Team, 2011, p. 5). However, as the cases in this volume show, at different stages of the research process (in the recursive cycle of generating ideas, planning, contributing and analysing data, learning, taking action, and generating new ideas) degrees of community participation may differ and change over time.

Ethical issues in research

This section discusses what we mean by 'ethical issues' and describes the growth of concern about ethics in research, outlining the main issues and how these are tackled in policy and practice through the growth of research governance systems. Following ordinary usage in English, we use the terms 'ethical' and 'moral' inter-changeably in this book.[1]

To put it simply, we use the term 'ethical issues' to encompass matters of harms, benefits, rights, duties, and responsibilities experienced by humans in relationship to each other and the ecosystem. What is identified or noticed as being harmful or a right, for example, varies between cultures and countries, and has changed over time.

Concerns regarding ethics in the context of research with 'human subjects' grew initially from responses to biomedical research conducted by doctors in Nazi Germany on people held in concentration camps during the Second World War (Mitscherlich & Mielke, 1949). This led to the Nuremberg Code (1949), present-ing 10 principles for medical research, the first of which was voluntary consent. This code shaped the Declaration of Helsinki, originally drafted in 1964 and most recently amended in 2013 (World Medical Association, 1964/2013), which out-lines the basic principles for medical research involving human subjects. Another later scandal with a major influence on the regulation of research was the Tuskegee Syphilis experiment in Alabama, USA. This involved denial of treatment to poor African American men with syphilis in order to allow medical researchers to study the long-term effects of the disease over a 40-year period, only ending in 1972 when the scandal broke (Reverby, 2000).

The main ethical issues raised by these and similar cases related to the need to prevent harm to the 'human subjects' involved in any research, ensuring that they were not exploited or physically or emotionally damaged. The importance of giving full information to people who were participating in experiments (or to their carers or proxies), treating them with dignity and respect, and gaining their informed consent came to be regarded as a *sine qua non* for ethically sound research. The Tuskegee scandal in the USA led to legislation and the establishment of a com-mission in 1974, which produced the very influential Belmont Report (National Commission for the Protection of Human Subjects of Biomedical and Behavioral Research, 1979). This report outlined three key ethical principles for research – respect for persons, beneficence, and justice – along with guidance regarding their

---

1 Some philosophers and other theorists distinguish 'morality' (concerned with societal norms) from 'ethics' (concerned with internally generated [personal] norms) (see Banks [2012, pp. 5–6] for further discussion).

application with respect to informed consent, assessment of risk and benefits, and selection of subjects.

These principles and guidelines are still highly influential, having come to dominate not only biomedical research, but also research in behavioural and social sciences. One criticism of this growth in regulatory ethics across the board is that there has been insufficient input from scholars in these latter disciplines (Schrag, 2010). Hence there is an over-emphasis on protection from harm and risk aversion, which does not necessarily fit with the circumstances of social research, let alone PR. This essentially 'top-down' approach is premised on a distinction between researcher and researched, assumes all research fits this ethical framework and reinforces systems of power and expertise which are actively challenged in PR. In recent years there has been a tendency to generate many more detailed rules and complex systems of research governance deriving from these principles, including ethical approval by review boards and committees, which can lull us into believing successfully completing an official form constitutes the end of our obligation to engage in ethical thinking and reflection (see Chapter 7 of this volume). Or as van den Hoonaard has wryly observed, 'paperwork, as we have seen, distracts committees from doing ethics work and researchers from pondering ethical considerations' (2011, p. 290).

In this book we provide an alternative ethical framework from the 'bottom up', which better reflects the realities and values of PR. This acknowledges the need to cultivate researchers with skills of good communication and relationship building, moral qualities of trustworthiness, honesty and care, and commitment to dialogue based on the nuances of the particular situations and people they encounter. We hope this volume, particularly the thoughtful and honest reflections provided by the case authors, will promote greater critical reflection on ethical issues in all research, and in PR in particular.

Ethical issues in participatory research

In designing the structure of the book we drew on a literature review undertaken as part of a scoping study coordinated by Durham University's Centre for Social Justice and Community Action (Durham Community Research Team, 2011). Common themes under which ethical challenges in PR might be grouped were outlined in Banks et al. (2013), of which the list below is a summary.

- *Partnership, collaboration and power* – all PR involves some degree of collaboration, whether between professional researchers and community partners or a range of different community researchers. Therefore it is important to attend to how partnerships are established, power distributed and control exerted. Ethical issues and dilemmas noted in the literature included: tackling mismatches between timelines and expectations of community organisations, funders and academics; awareness that closer research relationships also bring greater potential for exploitation; and acknowledging that co-researchers may experience moments of inclusion and exclusion in the research process.

- *Blurring the boundaries between researcher and researched, academic and activist* – insofar as PR involves some degree of co-production of research and an action-orientation, this may entail community members taking on roles of researchers, and professional researchers adopting roles commonly associated with health, social care or community development work. Tensions may arise for people who find themselves in the roles of both researcher and community advocate, or academic and activist. Community researchers studying their own communities or peer groups may play roles as both researchers and researched, and have to consider whether and where to draw lines between being researchers and friends or neighbours.

- *Community rights, conflict and democratic representation* – while most ethical codes and guidelines for research are concerned with rights of individual 'human subjects' (to safety, privacy, freedom of choice to participate or withdraw), PR in community-based settings raises the challenge of extending rights to communities or groups. This creates issues in defining 'community', taking account of conflict within and between communities and groups, and deciding who represents group or community interests. If the research topic is controversial, for example, attitudes towards assisted suicide amongst disabled people (see Minkler et al., 2002), complex matters relating to democracy and community relations have to be considered.

- *Ownership and dissemination of data, findings and publications* – if multiple partners are involved in research, there may be conflicts of interest regarding who takes credit for findings and what channels are used for dissemination. These may manifest themselves in decisions about co-authorship, publicity and claims for research impact, particularly with increasing academic pressures to publish and give evidence for impact on policy and practice.

- *Anonymity, privacy and confidentiality* – whilst these matters are common concerns in all social research, close relationships developed in PR preclude straightforward solutions. If community or peer researchers are involved, and wide dissemination is planned within the community, identities of research participants may be hard to conceal. Some participants may wish to be named and credited, others may not. There may be matters some representatives of a community or group do not wish to be revealed, such as survival strategies of asylum seekers, sex workers or indebted families.

- *Institutional ethical review processes* – a noticeable theme in the literature is the difficulty of fitting PR into the process and procedures for institutional ethical review (Brydon-Miller, 2009; Flicker & Guta, 2008; Love, 2011; Manzo & Brightbill, 2007). Whilst many assumptions underlying the ethical review process – including the predictability of research trajectories – are problematic for all social research, they pose specific challenges for PR. Ethical guidelines for research and forms to be completed are often premised on clear distinctions between researchers and subjects of research; require individual consent to participate; and make assumptions that an academic or professional researcher ('principal investigator') has primary control over, and responsibility for, the research.

These form the themes for Chapters 2–7 of the book. The topic for the final chapter (social action for social change) was suggested by one of the authors (Cathy Vaughan) as important in PR, which generally has a social change commitment that goes beyond simply creating 'impact':

- *Social action for social change* – The theoretical underpinnings of PR emphasise its action-orientation, as an approach to research that strives for social change. However what constitutes appropriate and sufficient 'action' is not always clear, with different partners holding varied views on what types of outcomes could be described as social action. That PR will involve social action is often assumed, with limited guidance available to research partners about the need to consider the nature of action, to plan for it and to reflect on where responsibility for this action lies. Research partners experience different constraints upon their social change efforts, including time, resources, control and institutional mandates.

While there is obvious overlap between these issues, we felt they provided a useful organising framework for the book. They are a mixture of ethical issues identified in 'traditional' (non-participatory) research (such as anonymity, privacy and confidentiality) and those that are more distinctive to PR (blurring boundaries, community rights and social action). Most cases were not written for a specific chapter in the book, so they give relatively holistic accounts of the research process and may raise issues relevant to the themes of several chapters.

Theoretical approaches to ethics[2]

So far we have described and categorised ethical issues in PR based on commonly accepted understandings of what counts as 'ethical'. We have said little about theories of ethics, particularly those emanating from moral philosophy, which tend to be concerned with identifying what lies at the heart of the 'good life', what counts as 'right', 'wrong', 'good' or 'bad', or what responsibilities humans have for each other and the ecosystem.

Such theories can be useful in offering frameworks within which to conceptualise ethical life, yet they can be also be problematic if we try to use them in making decisions and choices, as many ethical theories tend to focus on one feature of ethical life and it is often hard to link practice on the ground with high level theoretical systems. For example, on the basis of Kantian deontology, a key principle of

---

2 This section draws on Banks (2012).

right action is that each person should be respected as a unique individual, treated with dignity and never used as a means to an end (Baron, 1995; Kant, 1785/1964). Alternatively, according to utilitarianism, we decide what is right by calculating which course of action will promote the greatest well-being of the greatest number of people (Mill, 1863/1972; Singer, 2011). Both Kantianism and utilitarianism are theoretical systems based on universal ethical principles of right action, with decision-making based on impartial, rational deliberation.

Aristotelian virtue ethics, on the other hand, focuses attention first and foremost on the motives and moral qualities of human agents (the people doing the actions) as opposed to the actions themselves. According to Aristotle, the cultivation of virtuous character traits (such as respectfulness, courage, honesty, compassion) is essential for human flourishing (Aristotle, 350 BCE/1954; Snow, 2015). More recently the ethics of care has been developed, particularly (but not exclusively) by feminist philosophers, paying attention not just to people as moral agents, but above all to relationships between people and the responsibilities they have for each other based on their particular situations and contexts, such as mother and child (Held, 2006; Noddings, 1984). Other variations of more relational approaches to ethics include communitarian ethics, where the focus is less on the individual and more on the 'community', seeking solidarity, harmony and the common good (Gyekye, 2010; Kuczewski, 1997), and the 'ethics of proximity' based on the demand or call of the other person (Levinas, 1989; Løgstrup, 1997). These have resonances with covenantal ethics, as outlined by Hilsen (2006) and Brydon-Miller (2009) in the context of action research, which centres on the deep commitment, relationship of trust and unconditional responsibility between people, drawing on the religious notion of the covenant with God, redefined within the context of human relationships as 'community covenantal ethics'.

These relational approaches, particularly communitarian ethics, are much closer to those that are more prevalent in the global South and in Indigenous communities in the global North, where individuals are defined in relationship with others (Chuwa, 2014; Gbadegesin, 2005; Keown, 2005; Li, 1994). Virtue ethics, the ethics of care and communitarian ethics do not attempt to articulate universal abstract principles applying to all people, in all places, at all times. Rather they adopt a more situated (contextual) approach to ethics, starting from the realities of everyday life, as opposed to applying abstract principles. They regard emotions as an important feature of ethics, arguing that empathy and compassion, for example, are essential to ethical being and acting.

There are many other approaches to ethics that start with everyday practice, including narrative ethics, involving the use of stories to sharpen ethical sensibilities (Nelson, 1997) and case-based ethics (casuistry), which takes analysis of particular cases as a starting point, categorising and comparing them (Arras, 1991; Jonsen & Toulmin, 1988). These can more accurately be described as methodologies rather than theories, as they do not attempt to create normative theoretical systems based on foundational principles or concepts. Table 1.1 summarises these approaches to ethics in a simplified form.

TABLE 1.1: Some theoretical and methodological approaches to ethics (adapted from Banks, 2012, p. 10)

I. *Principle-based ethics* (ethical theories)
    a) *'Kantian' principles*, for example:
        • respect for persons as rational, self-determining beings;
        • impartiality and consistency in choice and action …

    b) *Utilitarian principles*, for example:
        • promotion of welfare/goods;
        • just distribution of welfare/goods …

II. *Character- and relationship-based ethics* (theoretical approaches)
    a) *Virtue ethics* – development of character/virtues/excellences, such as:
        • honesty;
        • compassion;
        • integrity …

    b) *Ethics of care* – importance of particular relationships, involving:
        • care;
        • attentiveness;
        • responsibility …

    c) *Communitarian ethics* – the primacy of community:
        • solidarity;
        • harmony;
        • inter-connectedness …

III. *Narrative and case-based ethics* (methodologies)

    a) *Narrative ethics* – collection of approaches that value and use stories:
        • listening to/reading stories to sharpen moral sensibilities;
        • telling stories to define and develop one's identity;
        • invoking stories as moral explanation …

    b) *Casuistry* – analysis of cases as a starting point, with a focus on:
        • specific circumstances of the case;
        • paradigm cases;
        • categorisation and comparison of cases …

Although these many ways of theorising about ethics, analysing cases and making ethical decisions may seem (and are sometimes presented by their proponents as) mutually exclusive, in fact they can usefully be regarded as complementary facets of a complete account of ethics. The idea of impartial principles of fairness and universally held rights and freedoms is an important way of looking at how people should be treated, especially in professional and international contexts. Principles provide a benchmark against which to assess decisions, actions and policies and highlight unjustified differences in treatment based on favouritism, prejudice, oppressive use of power and unfair legal, social and cultural laws, customs and norms. Our earlier discussion of the Nazi and Tuskegee experiments, which led to the development of principles for research ethics, are a case in point.

However, principle-based approaches do not capture all dimensions of what might be regarded as ethically important features of situations, especially in parts of the world or cultures where individual rights and freedoms have less prominence than family, group, tribe or community relationships and responsibilities. People's motives, character and emotions are also important, as are their particular relationships and responsibilities to each other and within their communities. Careful examination of specific features of each case or situation is vital, as is the ability to recognise morally relevant issues, compare with other cases and test against commonly accepted principles and rules. This capacity or quality is what Aristotle termed 'phronesis' ('practical wisdom'). It is a quality that needs to be nurtured and developed, through working alongside experienced role models or teachers, entailing the ability to notice, pay attention and see morally relevant features of situations (Banks, 2018b; Eikeland, 2008).

Attention to relationships and character is important in all realms of life, not just PR (see Banks, 2018a; Banks & Gallagher, 2009). Otherwise what we regard as the domain of ethics becomes very 'thin' – decontextualised from particular people and places. It is our view that the ethical domain is inseparable from other aspects of everyday life (the practical, technical and political). Although we necessarily abstract certain features from their contexts to compare and evaluate, it is important to start from details of the situations in which people are living and working, seeing ethics as deeply embedded in particular circumstances and embodied by people in their daily lives (Banks et al., 2013). Hence we regard cases (stories or narratives) as an invaluable aid to encouraging ethical sensitivity and reflective learning. This is particularly important in PR, which is a highly collaborative and relational practice, lending itself to theorising drawn from virtue, care and communitarian ethics, rather than abstract, universal principles.

Given our concern with particularities of situations, people and relationships, using narratives or cases is a useful methodology for developing ethical understanding. 'Casuistry' or case-based ethical reasoning (Jonsen & Toulmin, 1988) draws on a medieval Christian practice of providing moral guidance in particular situations. Rather than beginning with an ethical theory, casuistry starts with particular cases, taking account of the specific circumstances of each case in deciding on an ethically correct response. It works by taking a case and comparing it with a paradigm case, which is relatively straightforward and about which most people would agree in their ethical evaluations, determining differences and similarities. This is similar to legal reasoning, requiring skills in determining morally relevant features of cases and creating taxonomies of types of cases and issues. Casuistry is not a normative theory (prescribing what is good or bad), rather it is more akin to a method for making ethical assessments and decisions. In case-based ethics 'moral reasoning' plays a crucial role, with 'reasoning' in this sense including use of moral intuition and practical wisdom, as distinct from rationality based on abstract principles (Toulmin, 2001).

Since this book draws on cases from many different countries, this approach to ethical evaluation, starting with the case and pursuing a detailed and careful analysis, is very useful. Sometimes people who espouse very different ethical and religious values may come to agreement about what should be done in a particular case, by focusing on the details of the case. Their differences emerge when they come to justify their ethical evaluations with reference to different values or theories.

The nature of ethics cases and what we can learn from them

This book was conceived as a book of 'ethics cases'. In learning and teaching about practical ethics, it is common to use case examples as a way of encouraging students and practitioners to envisage how particular ethical challenges arise in practice and how they can be handled. It is less common to find longer real-life cases, extending over several pages, narrated by one or more key actors in the story, with a first person account of what they felt and thought, as well as what they did. The typical ethics case tends to be relatively short, often fabricated, told in the third person, focusing on action and encouraging the reader to consider what decision should be taken or to give an ethical evaluation of what happened (Banks, 2012; Chambers, 1997). The cases in this book are more diffuse, less focused on simply highlighting de-contextualised dilemmas, and more concerned to offer textured vignettes depicting key features of the characters, motives and emotions of the people involved, and the places and background circumstances germane to the stories. Of course, each case is written by an author or co-authors from a specific perspective, telling a particular story. That is what makes each story both a case and, specifically, an ethics case. A case is framed as an extract from a whole set of experiences, situations and incidents to tell a story that might make some sense to the reader as well as the teller. Since the authors were all asked to offer 'ethics cases', they have constructed them so as to foreground matters pertaining to ethics – issues relating to human well-being, harm, promotion or infringement of rights and responsibilities.

Collecting cases

The cases were collected over several years, inspired by projects on ethics in CBPR at Durham University in 2011–2012, which involved initially collecting UK-based cases (Banks & Armstrong, 2012). It was decided to expand the collection to include cases from around the world, inviting people through international conferences and networks to contribute. It became a project of the International Collaboration for Participatory Health Research in 2013, through which we made calls for cases. However, it was hard to get people to submit cases. Although relatively short compared with an article, a good case requires considerable work to tell a compelling story, clearly articulated, with the right amount of detail to give readers a good enough impression of the relevant circumstances, but not to overwhelm them. It also requires some courage – to expose authors' practice to scrutiny, particularly in cases where on reflection the authors wished the outcomes were different or they felt implicated in unethical practice. Even when cases ostensibly present the authors as 'hero/ines' or 'innocent victims', there is still a danger that readers will see other 'hidden' features and may call into question decisions and actions undertaken in good faith by the protagonists. Moreover, for this book, authors were asked to offer cases about which commentaries would be written by strangers, who knew nothing of them or their situations.

Our guidance to case authors included the following information:

> Cases usually focus on a particular situation or event that raised an ethical dilemma or problem for the person writing the case. They are usually written from the author's perspective and give an account of the issues as she/he saw them and may include reference to their feelings and thoughts.

> We are looking for cases about real situations, preferably written in the first person (that is, using 'I'). This should be a short description of a situation, an event or a piece of work – describing the important features. A case may describe everyday events and actions that an academic researcher, community researcher or other partner or participant encountered in practice that have ethical implications – or may be a description of a situation that is constructed as problematic – involving a difficult decision, a dilemma, or a situation where 'mistakes' were made.

Many of the cases were commissioned as a result of face-to-face contact at meetings and conferences. Others were gained through calls via the web or email, and a few were invited through correspondence with people we thought likely to have suitable material.

The balance between the global South and North

We made large efforts to commission cases from as many different countries as possible, but found it difficult to get as many as we would have liked from the global South. This reflects the limitations of our networks, and perhaps the fact that the request was written in English. Although we offered support with translation, it would be time-consuming to construct a case in English. It may also reflect the fact that 'ethics' and specifically 'research ethics' are topics that are well-defined and high on the agenda in the global North, but less so in the global South. This is not to say that issues of harms, benefits, rights and responsibilities are unimportant, but the concept of 'ethics' that abstracts these matters from everyday practical life is often less recognisable. Apparently, in some languages, for example in sub-Saharan Africa, there is no direct equivalent of the term 'ethics' (Gyekye, 2010). A concern with 'ethics' may be introduced, ironically, in the guise of regulatory practices as part of the research colonisation process of the global North.

Our argument in this book is that the impartial, detached approach to ethics that emphasises fairness and dominates the research ethics literature, policies and codes, is inadequate on its own as an ethical framework for PR, which is essentially a relational, embedded and embodied practice. This same argument applies to any kind of research or professional practice in many areas of the global South or Indigenous communities in the global North, where particular and partial human and ecological relationships and responsibilities are paramount. Hence Case 3.1, told by Pinky Shabangu, a community researcher working on an externally initiated project in Southern Africa, is particularly telling. She recounts her dilemma about whether to follow the research protocols stressed in her training (always asking everyone the same survey questions), as opposed to refraining from asking when she knows the answer (her informant's mother is dead), and she knows it will hurt the feelings of her informant (also a neighbour) to reply. Similarly, in Case 6.3, PhD researcher from Australia, Michelle Brear, recounts tensions between naming a group of community researchers from a southern African community at their request, and the condition of the Australian ethics committee approval based on maintaining anonymity. As Kalsem suggests in her commentary on this case, this would amount to the academic community, with its position and rules, getting the final say. Interestingly, between submitting the case and the completion of the final draft of the book, a decision was made to name some of the community researchers as co-authors of publications and the case was amended accordingly.

The focus of the cases

As readers will notice, the cases in the book are very varied in terms of:

- how much background information is given;
- the balance between descriptions of events and reflective accounts of cognitive and emotional processes;
- whether or not the account focuses on a specific problem or dilemma; and
- whether the author explicitly or implicitly invites readers to make their own evaluative judgements about what happened and what could have been done differently.

We (as editors) wanted to keep as close as possible to the original accounts and forms of expression of the case authors. However, in all cases we asked for further information and clarification about circumstances and actions. In some cases, particularly when the first language of the author was not English, we initiated some fairly substantial revisions, often over several iterations in dialogue with the case authors.

Degrees of participation

A few cases did not make it into the book as after discussion it became clear that the research was not what we judged to be 'participatory'. Indeed, a common question we asked several authors on receiving their first drafts was 'Can you explain how this research was participatory?'

Given there are so many different views about what exactly counts as 'participatory research' it is not surprising that this issue arose. Researchers may use participatory techniques (such as PhotoVoice or participatory mapping), but unless the people producing the photos or maps then go on to interpret their meaning in the context of the wider research project, then the extent to which the research can meaningfully be described as 'participatory' may be limited. In some cases the original intention of the initiating academic researcher was to be participatory in some stages of the research process, but the community researchers or other stakeholders were not interested in 'deep' participation. This was the situation described by Jenevieve Mannell in Case 2.3, as she reflects on her struggles to engage fully the community-based researchers with whom she was working in Rwanda:

> As an academic I value the idea of trying to bring about social change through my research consistent with a community-based participatory research epistemology, however for the local researchers involved in this project, research participation is just another piece of paid work.

This raises the well-known dangers of participation imposed from outside (Cooke and Kothari, 2001). In other cases, a research project may become more participatory than originally intended, as the initiating professional researchers realise what 'genuine' participation and power sharing with 'participants' or 'community researchers' could mean in practice. This happened in Case 2.4 as Candice Satchwell, the academic researcher, describes how she and her colleagues decided at the start of a project about young people's voices that they should involve young people as interviewers for the research assistant post.

Learning from mistakes

One of the matters on which we had to agree as editors was that these cases were not meant to be examples of 'best practice' – either in PR or handling ethical issues. They were designed as fairly honest accounts of what happens in everyday PR practice, which includes ethical infringements, wrong turns, mistakes and what might even be construed later by the case authors or readers as 'bad practice'. A significant number of cases end with reflective comments from the author wondering if they did the right thing, commenting on what they learnt and how they might act differently in the future. Doing 'good' PR, with a high degree of ethical sensitivity, takes time to learn. Learning by doing fits very much with a participatory epistemology (theory of knowledge), which values experiential as much as propositional and theoretical knowledge gained through reading books or listening to lectures (Heron & Reason, 2000). So, for example, in Case 3.2, Catherine Wilkinson describes how she thought it appropriate to become 'friends' with young people in a UK radio station where she was conducting PR. Towards the end of the case she offers this reflection:

> I suddenly began to question my entire approach to this participatory research project, which had drawn me into friendships with young people which I considered to be inevitable due to our comparable age, our liking of the same music, and our mutual interest in radio. I was left asking myself a series of questions: Is it ethical to build friendships with research participants?

Struggles for doctoral students

Wilkinson was a doctoral student, inevitably facing the challenges of inexperience and also having to meet certain criteria for writing a dissertation which contained her own work and reflections as well as the products of the collaborative research with young people. She undertook ethnographic research (observing young people in the radio station and interviewing them) as well as PR (working alongside them as researchers). Hence the young people were research subjects and informants as well as co-researchers, which added to the 'layering' and complexity of the relationships, as MacFarlane and Roche note in their commentary on this case in Chapter 3.

Several cases are about doctoral research (see Cases 3.2, 3.4, 4.1, 4.2, 5.1, 5.2, 5.4, 6.2, 6.3, 6.4, 7.2, 8.1, 8.3), often written by people looking back several years to the challenges they faced as students. Some of these authors give accounts of themselves as struggling, like Wilkinson, to work out their roles and how to position themselves in relation to co-researchers. For example, Duis (a doctoral researcher) and Baur in Case 8.1 recount how their original intention of acting as facilitators of social action amongst isolated women of Turkish and Moroccan origin in an urban neighbourhood in The Netherlands was modified to becoming advocates on behalf of the women. Finally they question their role altogether as it appeared that participation in the project was 'disempowering' for the women. Case 5.2, written by Wiebe, gives an account of her doctoral research with Indigenous young people in a heavily polluted industrial part of Canada. Not wanting to dominate or undertake 'extractive' research, Wiebe felt the young people should decide how to disseminate and use a film they made together documenting the environmental and social injustices of the area. However, at the point when Wiebe left, having completed her doctoral research, no decision had been made about dissemination, resulting in the documentary not being widely available. The issues described by these authors provide a reminder to those who mentor or supervise doctoral students to offer thoughtful and timely support as they attempt to negotiate these challenges.

The emergent nature of PR

All research is designed to generate 'new knowledge' and researchers expect (indeed may hope for) unanticipated findings. However, the process of conducting 'traditional' research is usually 'designed' in advance, with methods identified and a timescale of 'milestones' to be achieved along the way. In practice some of the detailed plans usually prove unrealistic in any research, but in PR unpredictability and 'messiness' are almost defining features (Brydon-Miller et al., 2003; Cook, 2009). This inevitably proves challenging for institutional review boards/research ethics committees, as outlined in Chapter 7, and can lead to unhelpful constraints on PR, when academic researchers do not feel able to change their original plans, or are wary of going back to review boards/ethics committees. The emergent nature of PR, and the need for flexibility and creativity on the part of the researchers involved, is a noticeable theme in many cases in this book. This is why PR can be particularly challenging for doctoral researchers, both due to their lack of research experience and the constraints of producing a doctoral dissertation to a timescale and in a prescribed format. The film produced by Wiebe and the young people in her doctoral research (Case 5.2) was unplanned, occurring at the end of the study period. Geralyn Hynes (Case 3.4), an academic researcher who was also a qualified nurse, realised during the course of a PhotoVoice project with people with respiratory conditions in an Irish hospital that she was, in fact, acting as a therapist as she worked with participants to make sense of their illness stories and their lives. This was not what she had expected, nor had participants signed up for 'conversations that exposed [their] deepest feelings'. Yet they found the experience positive. Hynes felt that an ethical review board would not look favourably on a project that was both a therapeutic intervention and research, so the therapeutic element remained 'covert'.

In research projects initiated by professional researchers, or by professional (academic) researchers and partner NGOs, who then seek people to act as co-researchers, there is no guarantee that people will sign up and if they do, they may not deliver what was anticipated or promised. There are several cases in the book where community researchers challenged academic researchers. For example, in Case 8.4 a researcher with feminist values working for an NGO on domestic violence finds one or two of the women community researchers expressing views with which she disagrees (blaming some women for the violence they experience). She then has to decide how to handle this – as a professional researcher (respecting the women's views), a domestic violence NGO worker (challenging the women) or as a friend driving the women home (having a creative conversation). These are not mutually exclusive. Deciding what to do in this case is not just a matter of picking a role and following a set of norms linked to that role. It involves sensitivity to the circumstances and feelings of the women, recognising the social and political milieux influencing their thinking, considering when and how to challenge (if a decision is made to challenge), and reflecting with co-workers at the NGO and other co-researchers. In short, it requires a considerable amount of cognitive and emotional work – the first stage of which is recognising there is an ethical issue in the first place.

Ethics work and everyday ethics

These cases depict their authors, along with their collaborators, undertaking cognitive, emotional and practical work. The authors give accounts of themselves striving to be sensitive to the feelings and views of others, reflecting on their identities as ethical researchers, questioning injustices, and reasoning about the right courses of action. Of course, these are retrospective accounts, written for a book on ethics in PR. So we would expect authors to construct cases telling some kind of ethical story and featuring themselves as moral agents. Nevertheless, the cases are interesting in that they reveal what the authors view as ethical issues (often focusing on everyday relationships) and how they give accounts of their reasoning and actions afterwards (showing themselves as ethically aware and reflective – in effect, performing through their writing as ethical agents). What the authors depict themselves doing in these cases, and what they are doing when writing the cases as reflective narratives, is a certain kind of moral labour, or what Banks (2016) calls 'ethics work', which refers to:

> the effort people put into seeing ethically salient aspects of situations, developing themselves as good practitioners, working out the right course of action and justifying who they are and what they have done.
>
> *(Banks, 2016, p. 35)*

Banks (2016) suggests that ethics work is a major component of 'everyday ethics' – a term that encapsulates a concern with the small everyday ongoing practices that influence how people treat each other and how they contribute to the well-being and harm of each other, broader society, and the environment. 'Everyday ethics' is premised on the idea ethics is about more than facing ethical dilemmas and making difficult decisions. It is about who we are as people (compassionate, just, wise, respectful) and our responsibilities to each other as inter-dependent, fellow human beings (see Banks et al. 2013 for a discussion of everyday ethics in CBPR).

A framework for ethical practice

We have argued that ethical practice in PR depends as much on the cultivation of good qualities of character and a sense of relational responsibilities as on applying abstract ethical principles or following rules. Nevertheless, a set of principles may serve as a useful framework to guide participatory researchers starting a project. The list of principles in Table 1.2 was developed by a group of UK community partners and academics, specifically with PR in mind. It has a relational focus, with the first principle being 'mutual respect' and subsequent principles very much reflecting the values of PR as described earlier (e.g. equality, democratic participation, collective action). This contrasts with the more individualistic focus of many codes of research ethics. Accompanying the statement of principles are practice guidelines covering practical matters such as working agreements, ownership of data, and so on.

TABLE 1.2 Ethical principles for community-based participatory research
(adapted from Centre for Social Justice and Community Action & National
Coordinating Centre for Public Engagement, 2012)

1. *Mutual Respect: developing research relationships based on mutual respect, including a commitment to:*
   • agreeing what counts as mutual respect in particular contexts.
   • everyone involved being prepared to listen to the voices of others.
   • accepting that people have diverse perspectives, different forms of expertise and ways of knowing that may be equally valuable in the research process.

2. *Equality and Inclusion: encouraging and enabling people from a range of backgrounds and identities (e.g. ethnicity, faith, class, education, gender, sexual orientation, (dis)ability, age) to lead, design and take part in the research, including a commitment to:*
   • seeking actively to include people whose voices are often ignored.
   • challenging discriminatory and oppressive attitudes and behaviours.
   • ensuring information, venues and formats for meetings are accessible to all.

3. *Democratic Participation: encouraging and enabling all participants to contribute meaningfully to decision-making and other aspects of the research process according to skill, interest and collective need, including a commitment to:*
   • acknowledging and discussing differences in the status and power of research participants, and working towards sharing power more equally.
   • communicating in language everyone can understand, including arranging translation or interpretation if required.
   • using participatory research methods that build on, share and develop different skills and expertise.

4. *Active Learning: seeing research collaboration and the process of research as providing opportunities to learn from each other, including a commitment to:*
   • ensuring there is time to identify and reflect on learning during the research, and on ways people learn, both together and individually.
   • offering all participants the chance to learn from each other and share their learning with wider audiences.
   • sharing responsibility for interpreting the research findings and their implications for practice.

5. *Making a Difference: promoting research that creates positive change for communities of place, interest or identity, including:*
   • engaging in debates about what counts as 'positive' change, including broader environmental sustainability as well as human needs or spiritual development, and being open to the possibility of not knowing in advance what making a 'positive difference' might mean.
   • valuing the learning and other benefits for individuals and groups from the research process as well as the outputs and outcomes of the research.
   • building a goal of positive change into every stage of the research.

TABLE 1.2 (Continued)

---

6. *Collective Action: individuals and groups working together to achieve change, including a commitment to:*
   - identifying common and complementary goals that meet partners' differing needs for the research.
   - working for agreed visions of how to share knowledge and power more equitably and promote social change and social justice.
   - recognising and working with conflicting rights and interests expressed by different interest groups, communities of practice or place.

7. *Personal Integrity: participants behaving reliably, honestly and in a transparent and trustworthy fashion, including a commitment to:*
   - working within the principles of community-based participatory research.
   - ensuring accurate and honest analysis and reporting of research.
   - being open to challenge and change, being flexible and prepared to work with conflict.

These principles, also available in an *Easyread* version with pictures (Centre for Social Justice and Community Action & National Coordinating Centre for Public Engagement, 2013) can be used at the start of a research partnership to help those involved develop a bespoke ethical framework for a piece of work (see Abma et al., 2019, Chapter 3). They can also inform institutional review boards and research ethics committees about ethical issues in PR, and provide support in teaching and learning – including when analysing and discussing some of the cases in this book in class.

Using this book

There are many ways this book can be used in learning and teaching, both with students studying PR, and practitioners wishing to develop their understanding and skills. Table 1.3 summarises some exercises that can be used (for further examples see Banks and Armstrong, 2012; Banks and Nøhr, 2012).

TABLE 1.3 Case-based exercises for use in learning and teaching

---

A. *Analysing a case.* Students/practitioners can be given a case from this book, without the accompanying commentary, and asked to discuss and analyse it in groups or individually. The following questions might be useful:

   1. What is your initial reaction to this case, including any feelings you might have about it?
   2. What are the ethical issues involved in this case?

TABLE 1.3 (continued)

3. What action would you take if you were the researcher(s)/practitioner(s) involved?
4. How would you justify this ethically?

B. *Writing a commentary.* Students/practitioners can be asked to write their own commentary on a case from the book, or one written by a colleague. The following points can be used as guidance:

1. *Audience.* Consider who will be the audience for your commentary and ensure you write in language the audience will understand.
2. *Ethical issues.* Highlight what you think are the key ethical issues in the case – how can they be understood?
3. *Reflection on context.* If you are from a different country than the country of the case, or a different area of work, you might like to reflect on similar issues in your own country or area of work – to what extent are these universal/general issues in a particular context?
4. *Think about how critical or judgemental you should be.* Consider how the author(s) of the case, or other people who feature in the case, might respond to your comments.
5. *Ending.* Finish the commentary with a conclusion, which could be your own position statement ('My opinion about this particular case is …' or 'at the heart of this problem lies ….') or a proposed solution to the problem or another suitable ending to the commentary.

C. *Writing a case example.* Students/practitioners with experience of PR could be asked to write a case example (about two pages) based on an ethically challenging situation they have faced, using the following guidelines:

1. *Background information.* Start with a short introduction about the context in which the case takes place – the setting, the people involved.
2. *Description of events, thoughts, feelings.* Describe what happened, including accounts of any thoughts or emotions and short reflections, if desired.
3. *Anonymity.* Consider whether the names of people, organisations and places should be changed and any identifying features removed or changed, in order to protect the identity of those involved.

D. *Other case-based exercises.* Cases or short vignettes about specific situations with ethical implications can also be used as the basis for other kinds of exercises. Here are two examples:

1. *Dilemmas cafés* – This method asks participants to offer cases for discussion in small groups in a safe, yet critical, group of peers. A guide for facilitators is available (Centre for Social Justice and Community Action, 2015).
2. *Participatory theatre* – short episodes from PR practice where an ethical transgression or experience of oppression has taken place can be used as the basis for groups of people to act out short scenarios, and then rehearse different options for action. A guide based on Boal's Theatre of the Oppressed is available (Banks et al., 2014).

Overview of the chapters

Having suggested some practical uses of the book, we will summarise each chapter, so readers may identify themes and cases of relevance to their particular interests.

Chapter 2: Partnership, collaboration and power. The Introduction by Groot and Abma discusses some of the challenges of partnership working in PR, including: establishing, sharing and exerting control and power; tackling the mismatch of timelines and expectations between partners; anticipating the risks associated with participation in PR; and ensuring sustainability of partnerships. Four cases are presented and discussed relating to: institutional challenges in conducting PR with older people nursing homes in Denmark; co-researching with people with Asperger's syndrome in the UK; tensions between community and university-based researchers working on gender-based violence in Rwanda; and including young people in a PR project in the UK. Commentaries on the cases are offered from two community co-researchers, alongside Groot and Abma.

Chapter 3: Blurring the boundaries between researcher and researched, academic and activist. In the introduction, McFarlane and Roche explore three inter-related tensions: challenges for community researchers regarding their 'insider' status as it clashes with the integrity of research methods; difficulties in social relationships between academic and community partners as they navigate personal and project boundaries; and dilemmas about unanticipated action and change. Four cases describe issues concerning: data collection on sensitive matters from people known to a community researcher in Southern Africa; relationships of friendship between a doctoral researcher and young people in a UK PR project; working with people with intellectual disabilities as co-researchers in Denmark; and recognising a PhotoVoice project with people in an Irish hospital as both research and therapy.

Chapter 4: Community rights, conflict, and democratic representation. This chapter engages questions regarding issues of power and privilege within and across communities involved in PR. In the introduction, speaking from her many years of conducting community-based research in marginalised communities in Bangladesh, Guhathakurta discusses issues of voice, positionality, intersectionality, and institutional power. These same themes are reflected in cases covering: work with temporary foreign workers in Canada; persons with disabilities in rural Zambia; Inuit and *Qallunaat* (non-Inuit) community workers in Artic Canada; and Roma and non-Roma residents of a 'socially excluded locality' in the Czech Republic.

Chapter 5: Co-ownership, dissemination and impact. In the introduction, Bos and Abma present an overview of ethical issues relating to: complexities of co-ownership; participatory dissemination; and ensuring social impact. Four cases are presented, focusing on: ethical disagreements over ownership of data and findings from community-based research in Tanzania; decolonising research through documentary film in Canada; conflicting realities between young service-users and policy-makers in Finland; and the meaning of 'co' in co-writing between an academic researcher and co-researcher with an intellectual disability in The Netherlands. Commentaries on the cases are offered from two community researchers, alongside Bos and Abma.

Chapter 6: Anonymity, privacy and confidentiality. The introduction examines anonymity, privacy and confidentiality from the perspective of a legal scholar and participatory researcher, Kristin Kalsem, providing a thoughtful framing of the ways in which these concepts—so often assumed in traditional research contexts—are problematised in PR. The cases deal with: breaches of confidentiality following the theft of project equipment in Canada; challenges faced by Canadian researchers working within an institutional setting in guarding privacy while insuring the participants are able to contribute to the research process; negotiating anonymity within the context of community-based participatory research in Swaziland in southern Africa; and supporting the rights of participants with disabilities in Vietnam to get credit for their contributions to the research process—both in local contexts as well as in the global arena of academic publishing.

Chapter 7: Institutional ethical review processes. Drawing upon experience as both community-based participatory researcher and ethical review board member, in the introduction to this chapter Guta reviews many challenges encountered in trying to understand and negotiate the specific issues PR presents, including conflicts of interest and coercion, the involvement of peer researchers, participant recruitment, and data management. Cases describe: issues raised for a research ethics committee chair when considering approval of a PR project relating to health care of migrants in Ireland; issues of parental consent for teenagers involved in a doctoral research project in the UK; concerns about participant burden and vulnerability in action research on palliative care in Ireland; and dilemmas in a UK PAR project involving mental health service users and providers.

Chapter 8: Social action for social change. In the introduction, Davis and Vaughan explore the action-orientation of PR by examining the relevant theoretical underpinnings, conceptualisations and impacts of power on action, and social change outcomes. A framework drawing on the ethics of reflexivity and solidarity is discussed as a means to maximise possibilities for action and change. Four cases cover issues relating to: challenges in trying to facilitate social action in a multi-ethnic neighbourhood in The Netherlands; how to ensure sustainability following PR on sexual and reproductive health of women with disabilities in the Philippines; researching for social change in rural livelihoods in a conservation area in rural South Africa; and conflicting views on socially just change in research on community-led responses to family violence in Australia.

We hope readers will find the material contributed by the many authors in this book as stimulating, educational and inspirational as we do.

References

Abma, T. A., Banks, S., Cook, T., Dias, S., Madsen, W., Springett, J., & Wright, M. (2019). *Participatory Research for Health and Social Well-Being*. Dordrecht, The Netherlands: Springer.

Aristotle. (350 BCE/1954). *The Nichomachean Ethics of Aristotle, translated by Sir David Ross.* London: Oxford University Press.

Arras, J. (1991). Getting Down to Cases: The Revival of Casuistry in Bioethics. *Journal of Medicine and Philosophy, 16* (1), 31–33.

Banks, S. (2012). Global Ethics for Social Work? A Case-based Approach. In S. Banks & K. Nøhr (Eds.), *Practising Social Work Ethics Around the World: Cases and Commentaries* (pp. 1–31). Abingdon: Routledge.

Banks, S. (2016). Everyday ethics in professional life: social work as ethics work, *Ethics and Social Welfare, 10*(1), 35–52.

Banks, S. (2018a). Cultivating resarcher integrity: Virtue-based approaches to research ethics. In N. Emmerich (Ed.), *Virtue Ethics in the Conduct and Governance of Social Science Research (Advances in Research Ethics and Integrity, Vol. 3)* (pp. 21–43). Bingley: Emerald Publishing.

Banks, S. (2018b). Practising professional ethical wisdom: The role of 'ethics work' in the social welfare field. In D. Carr (Ed.), *Cultivating Moral Character and Virtue in Professional Practices* (pp. 55–69). London: Routledge.

Banks, S., & Armstrong, A. (Eds.). (2012). *Ethics in community-based participatory research: Case studies, case examples and commentaries.* Durham and Bristol: Centre for Social Justice and Community Action and National Coordinating Centre for Public Engagement, available at: www.durham.ac.uk/socialjustice/ethics_consultation (accessed January 2018).

Banks, S., Armstrong, A., Carter, K., Graham, H., Hayward, P., Henry, A., . . . Strachan, A. (2013). Everyday ethics in community-based participatory research. *Contemporary Social Science, 8*(3), 263–277.

Banks, S., & Butcher, H. (2013). What is community practice? In S. Banks, H. Butcher, A. Orton, & J. Robertson (Eds.), *Managing Community Practice: Principles: Policies and Programmes, 2nd edition* (pp. 7–30). Bristol: Policy Press.

Banks, S.,& Gallagher, A. (2009). *Ethics in professional life: Virtues for health and social care.* Basingstoke: Palgrave Macmillan.

Banks, S., Hart, A., Pahl, K., & Ward, P. (2019). Co-producing research: a community development approach. In S. Banks, A. Hart, K. Pahl, & P. Ward (Eds.), *Co-producing research: A community development approach* (Chapter 1). Bristol: Policy Press.

Banks, S. & Nøhr, K. (Eds.). (2012). *Practising Social Work Ethics Around the World: Cases and Commentaries.* Abingdon: Routledge.

Banks, S., Rifkin, F., Davidson, H., Holmes, C., & Moore, N. (2014). *Performing ethics: Using participatory theatre to explore ethical issues in community-based participatory research.* Durham, UK: Centre for Social Justice and Community Action, Durham University, www.durham.ac.uk/socialjustice/ethics_consultation/ (accessed January 2018).

Baron, M. (1995). *Kantian Ethics Almost Without Apology*. Ithaca, NY: Cornell University Press.

Bivens, F., Haffenden, J., & Hall, B. (2015). Knowledge, Higher Education and the Institutionalization of Community-University Research Partnerships. In B. Hall, R. Tandon, & C. Trembley (Eds.), *Strengthening Community University Research Partnerships: Global Perspectives* (pp. 5–30). Victoria, Canada: University of Victoria.

Brydon-Miller, M. (2009). Covenantal ethics and action research: Exploring a common foundation for social research. In D. Mertens & P. Ginsberg (Eds.), *Handbook of social research ethics* (pp. 243-258). Newbury Park, CA: SAGE.

Brydon-Miller, M., Greenwood, D., & Maguire, P. (2003). Why action research? *Action Research, 1*(1), 9–28.

Centre for Social Justice and Community Action. (2015). *Dilemmas cafés: a guide for facilitators*. Durham: Centre for Social Justice and Community Action, Durham University, available at: www.durham.ac.uk/socialjustice/ethics_consultation (accessed January 2018).

Centre for Social Justice and Community Action & National Coordinating Centre for Public Engagement. (2012). *Community-based participatory research: A guide to ethical principles and practice*. Bristol: NCCPE, available at: www.durham.ac.uk/socialjustice/ethics_consultation (accessed January 2018).

Centre for Social Justice and Community Action & National Coordinating Centre for Public Engagement. (2013). *Doing research together: How to make sure things are fair and no one is harmed*. Durham: Centre for Social Justice and Community Action, available at www.durham.ac.uk/socialjustice/ethics_consultation (accessed January 2018).

Chambers, R. (1994). The origins and practice of participatory rural appraisal. *World Development, 22*(7), 953–969.

Chambers, T. (1997). What to Expect from an Ethics Case (and What it Expects from You). In H. Nelson (Ed.), *Stories and their limits: narrative approaches to bioethics* (pp. 171–184). New York and London: Routledge.

Chuwa, L. T. (2014). *African Indigenous Ethics in Global Bioethics: Interpreting Ubuntu*. New York: Springer.

Cooke, B., & Kothari, U. (Eds.). (2001). *Participation: the new tyranny?* London: Zed.

Cook, T. (2009). The purpose of mess in action research: Building rigour though a messy turn. *Educational Action Research, 17*(2), 277–291.

Coughlin, S., Smith, S., & Fernandez, M. (2017). *Handbook of Community-Based Participatory Research*. New York: Oxford University Press.

Crow, C., & Allan, G. (1994). *Community Life: An introduction to local social relations*. Hemel Hempstead: Harvester Wheatsheaf.

Durham Community Research Team. (2011). *Community-based Participatory Research: Ethical Challenges*. Durham: Centre for Social Justice and Community Action, Durham University, www.durham.ac.uk/socialjustice/researchprojects/cbpr/ (accessed January 2018).

Eikeland, O. (2008). *The ways of Aristotle: Aristotelian philosophy of dialogue, and action research* (Studies in Vocational and Continuing Education, Vol. 5). Berlin: Peter Lang.

Fals Borda, O. (1987). The application of Participatory Action-Research in Latin America. *International Sociology, 2*(4), 329–347.

Fals Borda, O. (1988). *Knowledge and People's Power: Lessons with Peasants in Nicaragua, Mexico and Colombia*. New Delhi: Indian Social Institute.

Fals Borda, O. (2001). Participatory (action) research in social theory: Origins and challenges. In P. Reason & H. Bradbury (Eds.), *Handbook of action research: Participative inquiry and practice* (pp. 27–37). London: SAGE.

Fals Borda, O., & Rahman, M. (1991). *Action and knowledge: Breaking the monopoly with participatory-action research* New York: The Apex Press.

Flicker, S., & Guta, A. (2008). Ethical Approaches to Adolescent Participation in Sexual Health Research. *Journal of Adolescent Health, 42*(1), 3–10.

Freire, P. (1972). *The Pedagogy of the Oppressed*. London: Penguin.

Gaventa, J. (1993). The powerful, the powerless, and the experts: Knowledge struggles in an information age. In P. Park, M. Brydon-Miller, B. Hall, & T. Jackson (Eds.), *Voices of change: Participatory research in the United States and Canada* (pp. 21–40). Westport, CT: Bergin and Garvey Press.

Gbadegesin, S. (2005). Origins of African Ethics. In W. Schweiker (Ed.), *The Blackwell Companion to Religious Ethics* (pp. 413–422). Oxford: Blackwell.

Gyekye, K. (2010). African Ethics *Stanford Encyclopedia of Philosophy*: http://plato.stanford. edu/entries/african-ethics/ (accessed December 2010).

Hall, B. (1975). Participatory Research: An Approach for Change. *Convergence, 8*(2), 24–32.

Hall, B. (2005). In From the Cold? Reflections on Participatory Research From 1970–2005. *http://www.participatorymethods.org/resource/cold-reflections-participatory-research-1970–2005* (accessed January 2018).

Hall, B., & Tandon, R. (2018). From action research to knowledge democracy: Cartagenia 1997–2017. *Revista Colombiana de Sociología, 41*(1), 227–236.

Held, V. (2006). *The Ethics of Care: Personal, Political, and Global.* Oxford: Oxford University Press.

Heron, J., & Reason, P. (2000). The practice of cooperative inquiry: research 'with' rather than 'on' people. In P. Reason & H. Bradbury (Eds.), *Handbook of Action Research* (pp. 179–188). London: SAGE.

Hilsen, A. I. (2006). 'And they shall be known by their deeds': Ethics and politics in action. Action Research, *4*(1), 23–36.

Horton, B. (1993). The Appalachian land ownership study: Research and citizen action in Appalachia. In P. Park, M. Brydon-Miller, B. Hall, & T. Jackson (Eds.), *Voices of change: Participatory research in the United States and Canada* (pp. 85–102). Westport, CT: Bergin and Garvey Press.

International Collaboration for Participatory Health Research (ICPHR). (2013). *Position Paper No. 1: What is Participatory Health Research?* Berlin: ICPHR, www.icphr.org/ position-papers (accessed January 2018).

Jonsen, A., & Toulmin, S. (1988). *The Abuse of Casuistry: A History of Moral Reasoning.* Berkeley: University of California Press.

Kant, I. (1785/1964). *Groundwork of the Metaphysics of Morals,* trans H. Paton. New York: Harper and Row.

Keown, D. (2005). Origins of Buddhist Ethics. In W. Schweiker (Ed.), *The Blackwell Companion to Religious Ethics* (pp. 286–296). Oxford: Blackwell.

Kuczewski, M. (1997). *Fragmentation and Consensus: Communitarian and Casuist Bioethics.* Washington, D.C.: Georgetown University Press.

Levinas, E. (1989). Ethics as First Philosophy, translated by Seán Hand. In S. Hand (Ed.), *The Levinas Reader* (pp. 75–87). Oxford: Blackwell.

Li, C. (1994). The Confucian Concept of *Jen* and the Feminist Ethics of Care: A Comparative Study. *Hypatia: A Journal of Feminist Philosophy, 9*(1), 70–89.

Løgstrup, K. (1997). *The Ethical Demand.* Notre Dame, IN: University of Notre Dame Press.

Love, K. (2011). Little known but powerful approach to applied research: community-based participatory research. *Geriatric Nursing, 32*(1), 52–54.

Maguire, P. (1987). *Doing participatory research: A feminist approach.* Amherst, MA: The Center for International Education.

Manzo, L., & Brightbill, N. (2007). Towards a participatory ethics. In S. Kindon, R. Pain, & M. Kesby (Eds.), *Participatory action research approaches and methods: connecting people, participation and place* (pp. 33–40). Abingdon: Routledge.

Merrifield, J. (1993). Putting scientists in their place: Participatory research in Environmental and occupational health. In P. Park, M. Brydon-Miller, B. Hall, & T. Jackson (Eds.), *Voices of change: Participatory research in the United States and Canada* (pp. 65–84). Westport, CT: Bergin and Garvey Press.

Mill, J. S. (1863/1972). *Utilitarianism, On Liberty, and Considerations on Representative Government,* London: Dent.

Minkler, M., Fadem, P., Perry, M., Blum, K., Moore, L., & Rogers, J. (2002). Ethical dilemmas in participatory action research: a case study from the disability community. *Health Education and Behaviour, 29*(1), 14–29.

Mitscherlich, A., & Mielke, F. (1949). *Doctors of infamy: the story of the Nazi medical crimes.* New York: Schuman.

National Commission for the Protection of Human Subjects of Biomedical and Behavioral Research. (1979). *The Belmont Report: Ethical principles and guidelines for the protection of human subjects of research.* Washington, DC: Department of Health, Education and Welfare, www.hhs.gov/ohrp/regulations-and-policy/belmont-report/read-the-belmont-report/index.html (accessed January 2018).

Nelson, H. (Ed.) (1997). *Stories and their limits: narrative approaches to bioethics.* New York and London: Routledge.

Noddings, N. (1984). *Caring: A Feminine Approach to Ethics and Moral Education.* Berkeley and Los Angeles: University of California Press.

Park, P., Brydon-Miller, M., Hall, B., & Jackson, T. (Eds) (1993). *Voices of change: Participatory research in the United States and Canada.* Westport, CT: Bergin and Garvey Press.

Plant, R. (1974). *Community and Ideology.* London: Routledge and Kegan Paul.

Reason, P., & Bradbury, H. (2008). Introduction. In P. Reason & H. Bradbury (Eds.), *The SAGE Handbook of Action Research: Participative Inquiry and Practice* (pp. 1–10). London: SAGE.

Reverby, S. (Ed.) (2000). *Tuskegee's truths: Rethinking the Tuskegee syphilis study.* Chapel Hill: University of North Carolina Press.

Schrag, Z. M. (2010). *Ethical imperialism: Institutional review boards and the social sciences, 1965–2009.* Baltimore, MD: The Johns Hopkins University Press.

Singer, P. (2011). *Practical Ethics, 3rd edition.* Cambridge: Cambridge University Press.

Smith, L. (1999). *Decolonizing Methodologies: Research and Indigenous Peoples.* London: Zed Books.

Snow, N. (Ed.) (2015). *Cultivating Virtue: Perspectives from Philosophy, Theology, and Psychology.* Oxford: Oxford University Press.

Somerville, P. (2016). *Understanding Community: Politics, Policy and Practice, 2nd edition.* Bristol: Policy Press.

Swantz, M.-L. (1974). *Participant Role of Research in Development (unpublished paper).* Dar es Salaam, Tanzania: Bureau for Resource and Land Use Productivity, University of Dar es Salaam.

Tandon, R. (Ed.) (2005). *Participatory research: Revisiting the roots.* New Delhi: Mosaic Books.

Thomas, T. and Narayanan, P. (2015) Introduction: powering knowledge from the margins. In T. Thomas and P. Narayanan (Eds) *Participation Pays. Pathways for post-2015* (pp. 1–4). Rugby, UK: Practical Action Publishing.

Toulmin, S. (2001). *Return to Reason.* Cambridge, MA: Harvard University Press.

van den Hoonaard, W. C. (2011). *The seduction of ethics: Transforming the social sciences.* Toronto: University of Toronto Press.

Wallerstein, N., Duran, B., Oetzel, J., & Minkler, M. (Eds.). (2017). *Community-Based*

Participatory Research for Health: Advancing Social and Health Equity, 3rd Edition. San Francisco: Jossey Bass.

World Medical Association. (1964/2013). *WMA Declaration of Helsinki – Ethical Principles for Medical Research Involving Human Subjects,* https://www.wma.net/what-we-do/medical-ethics/declaration-of-helsinki/ (accessed January 2018).

2

PARTNERSHIP, COLLABORATION AND POWER

Barbara Groot and Tineke Abma

With cases contributed by Annette Bilfeldt, Jackie Robinson, Jenevieve Mannell and Candice Satchwell, and additional commentaries by Melanie Peterman and Ruud Van Zuijlen

PART 1: INTRODUCTION AND OVERVIEW OF THE ISSUES

Barbara Groot and Tineke Abma

Important and complex: the world of partnership, collaboration and power

This chapter discusses the challenges participatory researchers experience in developing and maintaining partnerships, working together collaboratively and negotiating power relations. This is one of the most important, yet also complex and difficult, aspects of participatory research. In this chapter introduction we offer an overview of some of the issues raised in the literature on this topic and how these relate to the four cases in the second part of the chapter.

Participatory research involves multiple partners working together. In the field of health and social well-being, research groups may include engaged citizens, service user and patient experts, professionals from service user/patient organisations, health and social welfare professionals, directors and researchers from health organisations, academic researchers and policy-makers. But how do all those people and organisations establish working relationships? How do they develop and maintain partnerships? How do they deal with power? What do they think is 'good' collaboration? In the 'rush' of conducting participatory research we sometimes forget to take enough effort and time to reflect on, and act thoughtfully in relation to, these very important questions.

For some people the term 'partnership' may have connotations of legal, formal, written agreements. However, in the context of participatory research, particularly community-based participatory research, the term 'partnership' is used in a very broad sense to cover all kinds of relationships, both formal and informal. And usually these are 'collaborative' relationships, involving people working together to achieve shared goals. Such relationships involve 'building and maintaining trust', 'reading each other', 'seeing each other as persons' and 'connecting'. Central to our vision of collaboration is being open-minded, listening, taking each other seriously, giving room for everyone's capabilities and giving support when necessary. Although some research partnerships may involve a written agreement or contract (especially if a university is involved and finances and responsibilities have to be allocated among different organisations), the most important feature of a partnership is that it involves a dialogical, respectful and valued relationship, rather than a (written) contract.

In the next section of this chapter we give an overview of some key ethical challenges facing participatory researchers concerning 'partnership, collaboration and power' as recounted in the academic literature. This topic is well-discussed. It is one of the main themes of a recently published systematic review (Wilson et al., 2018) and was also identified as a theme in several reviews about ethical challenges in participatory research (Banks et al., 2013; Boser, 2007; Brydon-Miller, 2012; Mikesell et al., 2013; Souleymanov et al., 2016). We will discuss the following core ethical questions about responsibilities:

1) Establishing, sharing and exerting control and power.
2) Tackling the mismatch of timelines and expectations between partners.
3) Anticipating the risks associated with participation in participatory research.
4) Ensuring sustainability of the participatory research partnerships.

For each theme we give a summary of the issues, why these occur in participatory research and how participatory researchers can handle them.

After the overview of the literature in Part 1, four cases from different places around the world are presented in Part 2 (Denmark, Australia, UK/Rwanda and the UK). The cases present ethical challenges within different contexts, including rural Western and African communities, and with various priority groups, ranging from older people to people with Asperger's syndrome to young people. Following each case there is a commentary, compiled from discussions between Melanie Peterman and Ruud van Zuijlen (community-based researchers with experience of disability) and Tineke Abma and Barbara Groot (academic researchers). All four of us are white Dutch and have worked together in participatory research for three years as partners in a Community of Practice on participation and participatory research in the Centre of Client Experience (www.centrumvoorclientervaringen. com). Melanie has had paraplegia since 2002, while Ruud has been dealing with Multiple Sclerosis (MS) since he was a student. They have been working as 'patient experts' for 10 and 30 years respectively. Tineke and Barbara work in the academy. Barbara is a PhD student, researching the topic of collaboration in participatory research and Tineke is Professor of Participation and Diversity at VU University Medical Centre in Amsterdam.

Ethical issues related to partnership, collaboration and power

1) Who establishes, shares and controls power?

Participatory research holds the potential to democratise and decolonise knowledge production by engaging a wide range of people as partners in research, including those whose voices are seldom heard and who are often classified as 'vulnerable' or 'hard to reach'. In practice, control of research by people whose lives are the subject of the study and/or equal partnerships between 'professional' and 'community' researchers is much less common than professional control with elements of participation by community partners. The balance of power may change over time and across different aspects of the research when partnerships are established (Durham Community Research Team, 2011).

People whose lives or work are the subject of the study are often assigned multiple, ambiguous subject positions (Janes, 2016), for example: 'participant', 'partner-stakeholder', 'insider', 'peer', 'co-researcher', 'community researcher' or 'volunteer'. Researchers from universities are mostly identified as 'academic researcher', 'outsider researcher', 'university-based researcher' or 'professional researcher'. For all researchers, it is important to ask questions about: how we identify ourselves; whether others have the right to identify themselves; how we denominate our positions and the positions of all involved; and whether we confirm power differences in naming and assigning the positions in the research team?

In participatory research, facilitating shared decision-making processes and ways to discuss sharing and controlling power are key issues. But how can we facilitate this in an appropriate and 'good' way? Who is involved in decisions? Does everybody need to be involved in every decision? Who is in the lead? Who takes the final decision? How do we deal with the differential power of all partners in this decision-making process (Kuriloff et al., 2011)? Other questions are: Who initiates a project? Who makes decisions about who is working (paid or on a voluntary basis) in the research and who is not? Is everyone willing to share power and resources? A final question about responsibility and sustainability is: what responsibilities do, for example, academic partners have in ensuring financial compensation for the efforts of the people whose lives are the subject of the study beyond the span of the research project (Puffer et al., 2013)?

Basically, the underlying question is whether we start from a domination model with the usual hierarchies and authorities based on positions and ranking, or whether we work from a more egalitarian partnership model based on mutual, caring relationships? In all the four cases later in this chapter this question is very important. In Case 2.1, a university researcher is confronted with hierarchy in a partner organisation and its effect on the collaboration. The authors of Cases 2.2, 2.3 and 2.4 all reflect on their own power to make decisions and their roles in their participatory research practice.

Why do these challenges occur?

Participatory research starts from a commitment to involve a variety of partners, sharing power and resources, working from a position that is based on social justice premises and seeks beneficial outcomes for all participants. Working from these principles, a wide range of complex ethical issues arises (Banks et al., 2013). Reasons for these challenges include: there are often mixed groups of partners belonging to various social categories; there are power differences between the partners; and there is a tension between 'system' and 'life-world' (Habermas, 1987).

Participatory researchers almost inevitably have to reflect on issues of power, because being critical of irrationalities, inhuman situations and social injustice is the heart of participatory research (Kemmis, 2008). Reflections include power issues, as Lincoln (2009, p. 152) sums up, 'between persons, and power relations connected to institutions, historical circumstances, economics, gender, social location, race, class, sexual orientation, cultural backgrounds and experiences and actual location'. In addition, partners in participatory research differ in other respects, including educational level, legal status, health status, cognitive ability, language preference and/or membership in stigmatised groups (Mertens & Ginsberg, 2008). Most groups comprise academics and non-academics, paid and volunteer staff, people who are employed or unemployed, and professionals from different (hierarchical) professions. A participatory researcher who strives to facilitate a shared decision-making process, is confronted with privileges, disadvantages and related power dynamics. Especially if funders of the research or policy-makers are involved actively in research, it enlarges the political nature of the work. Working together with people who can make impactful decisions for those involved could increase tensions in collaboration.

In addition the attitude of the different partners can also create tensions. Tensions can arise from 'differing expectations, assumptions and agendas of community and academic partners that involve conflicting beliefs about research aims and outcomes' (Mikesell et al., 2013). Some partners, for example, have misguided perceptions of academic researchers' roles, especially if a participatory research project is academic-led or -initiated. The researchers, for example, might be seen to benefit the most from research involvement (Minkler, 2004). Despite good intentions, power and privilege associated with researchers working in the academy also make it difficult to develop relationships and trust in response to injustices (Brabeck et al., 2015). Moreover, non-academics often participate on a voluntary basis or for little reimbursement, 'providing free labour to support the research enterprise' (Brunger & Wall, 2016).

These tensions could as well be analysed from the perspective of Habermas (1987) and his theory of differences between the 'system' and 'life-world'. Habermas argues that the 'life-world' is based on communication, agreement and consensus, while the 'system' concentrates on economy, bureaucracy, market and state (Habermas, 1987). Funders, academic researchers and professionals work in a cost-benefit system logic where efficiency, productivity and utility are the driving forces. Strategic action is the common way to communicate, and this may conflict with the 'life-world' and the reproduction of cultural values, meaning and motivation and communicative action. System logics can hinder working according to the principles of participatory research. Yet, while funders, academics and partners have to align with the system, for people whose lives are the subject of the study, without an academic background, the system is not easily accessible. Writing proposals for funding agencies is problematic because of difficult formats, tight deadlines and conditions that may even hinder a good start. Besides, in research proposals funders are keen on descriptions that justify hours spent on achieving pre-described outcomes. This does not (at all) promote patient or community participation or power-sharing with the 'target group' in research. It may lead to alienation. Moreover, most academic organisations are not yet flexible in assigning paid jobs at the university to people without certificates. There are also many challenges faced by participatory research studies as they are assessed by academic review boards of positivistic medical research institutes (Fouché & Chubb, 2017). These are just a few examples.

How can we handle these challenges?

There are no easy answers or sets of rules about how to handle the issues of establishing, sharing and controlling power. An awareness of the potential complexities and conflicts and a willingness and ability amongst all research partners to critically reflect together on such issues throughout the planning are very important (Banks et al., 2013; Souleymanov et al., 2016; Bainbridge, 2013). In particular, Kuriloff and colleagues (2011) advise that researchers should develop an 'ethical stance', seeing every decision in the process as an ethical one that could affect the lives of people involved. This requires much more time to work on one's own ethical development, for example reading about ethics and PAR (Kuriloff et al., 2011). Others, such as Shore (2006) stress the potential of feminist ethics, an approach to analysing the power dynamics in research. Besides acknowledgement of positions of power and vulnerability, feminist ethics accounts for structural factors.

Acting ethically is not just the responsibility of academic researchers. As noted previously, a critical reflective stance with partners helps in discussing the issues. Training about research methods, especially together with a range of partners (Banks et al., 2013; Mikesell et al., 2013) could help in dealing with dilemmas and opening conversations about challenges from all perspectives. Putting ethics on the training agenda helps to reconcile difficulties.

Finally, an important piece of advice given in the literature is to be aware of the political nature of this work. Participatory research facilitators work in a politically strategic arena, which requires that they are skilled and comfortable to work through conflict (Shore, 2006). Reflecting in first person inquiry (Reason & Torbert, 2001) about leadership and mutual power, can help a facilitator enhance their skills in 'Developmental Action Logics' (Torbert, 2003, 2004). For example, the facilitator may start as a 'diplomat', who provides 'social glue' in the group and ensures that attention is paid to the interests and needs of others, and move to the role of 'strategist', who 'masters the second-order' impact of actions and agreements and the 'social interplay between personal relationships, organizational relations, and national and international developments' (Rooke & Torbert, 2005).

2) Dealing with the mismatch of timelines and expectations between partners

As noted before, tensions between partners can arise from differing expectations, assumptions and agendas, with conflicting beliefs about research aims and outcomes (Mikesell et al., 2013), timelines, research methodology (Banks et al., 2013; Minkler, 2004) and compensation for participation (Bainbridge, 2013). This could lead to questions like: How do we deal with all these expectations? Is it a good idea to have one or more people act as research facilitator(s), and if so, what are their roles? How much room do the facilitators have to take time and effort to explore expectations and reflect on them?

Below we offer a few examples of common mismatches in participatory research. People whose lives are the subject of the study sometimes 'expect more immediate results than can realistically be achieved' (Walsh et al., 2008). Substantial time lapses between initial engagement of people whose lives are the subject of the study and funding is often a reality. Non-academic partners are not 'accustomed to the numerous steps involved with research protocols and can become frustrated over the long process' (Love, 2011). The analysis phase of the research may be time-consuming, and not yet action-oriented. Furthermore, participatory research studies often work with small budgets (Ochocka et al., 2002; Bainbridge, 2013). Non-academic partners could have expectations about providing resources for people interviewed or purchasing equipment (Bainbridge, 2013). Finally, people whose lives are the subject of the study could be disappointed about unreasonable timeframes for remunerating people's effort in the research. Simple practical arrangements, for example organising financial reimbursement, could take a huge effort for an academic who works in a system that is not accustomed to participatory research studies (Bainbridge, 2013). This could leave a mark on relations and could lead to declining interest and engagement (Bainbridge, 2013) and even give feelings of stress (Ochocka et al., 2002).

The author of Case 2.3 describes a typical example of the mismatch of expectations of participation written in a research funding proposal and the real world in which participation is just a piece of paid work.

Why do these challenges occur?

Mismatches may occur because of partners' lack of knowledge and experience in adhering to research protocols (O'Neill et al., 2012; Salmon, et al., 2010; Smith, et al., 2008). Besides, academic researchers are often stuck in two worlds. One is the system in which funders, universities and academic boards ask researchers to work with deadlines, funding time schedules, fixed small budgets arranged to organise prescribed outcomes, and financial and personnel administration. The other is the life-world in which academics work together with community partners and see people experiencing vulnerable situations and social injustice, and are aware of the eagerness of the community partners to change their situations. Research facilitators are often in between both worlds, which means they have to deal with all the clashes and conflicts.

How can we handle these challenges?

It is not easy to enhance knowledge about participatory research in a short period. Zooming into the expectations about timelines and being proactive in planning research tasks, such as the ethics board application (Walsh et al., 2008) is a beginning. Putting the topic 'timelines' on the agenda of every partnership group meeting creates more realistic expectations (Ochocka et al., 2002).

Moreover, it takes time for facilitators to find their way in the 'interference' zone between the system and life worlds (Abma et al., 2017). Openness and dialogue about the different worlds and dilemmas are ways to create understanding back and forth (Love, 2011). Drawing on theory, the role of facilitator requires the skills and a philosophy of 'servant leadership' (Greenleaf, 1977). Servant leaders combine their motivation to lead with the need to serve, they express humility, authenticity, interpersonal acceptance and stewardship and provide direction for the group. Trust, fairness and a high-quality relationship are important for servant leadership (Van Dierendonck, 2011). Servant leadership is about going 'beyond one's self-interest', with the will in the first place to serve, and in the second place to lead (Greenleaf, 1977).

3) How can we be aware of the risks associated with participating in participatory research?

In participatory research we do not talk about the 'research population' or 'respondents' as in positivistic science. People who are actively involved in participatory research are often called and, perceived as, 'partners', 'co-researchers' or 'co-creators'. This difference brings some risks and vulnerabilities, foremost to the people whose lives are the subject of the study. Particularly because participatory research often focusses on sensitive topics and enters 'the social space generally barred to outsiders' (Dodson et al., 2007), it raises serious ethical issues. In the literature this topic is not yet broadly documented, although there are some writings about ethical dilemmas in research with undocumented citizens (Dodson et al., 2007; Letiecq & Schmalzbauer, 2012). In practice risks for people whose lives are the subject of the study are top of the mind in participatory research and this is not limited to undocumented people. People that rely on care or support, or stigmatised groups, could also be at risk by participating in participatory research. For example, their stories or criticisms of the care and support they receive might be traced and used to sanction them. Participation can then become disempowering (Kemmis & McTaggart, 2005).

Sharing personal sensitive stories and photographs could be a risk to peoples' personal and family lives, their community or peers. People may not be able to foresee the impact of sharing a personal story. Researchers may have to deal with disclosures reflecting practices of everyday illegality, which raises questions about how much should be represented and criticised. A breach of confidentiality in research could have disastrous consequences for people, such as being sent out of the country, losing critical resources or losing their children (Dodson et al., 2007; Letiecq & Schmalzbauer, 2012). It could also have negative consequences for people like them, because prejudices against certain groups of people could be deepened and mistrust of groups in society might rise (Achkar & Macklin, 2009; Brabeck et al., 2015). Research could reinforce stereotyped images of people, including malign versions of low-income people and people of colour (Dodson & Schmalzbauer, 2005). Illegal practices that are survival strategies for people living in vulnerable situations could get more attention. This could risk their lives, and also those of their peers (Dodson et al., 2007).

In Case 2.2, Jackie Robinson describes her concerns about the risks for the co-researchers (who have Asperger's syndrome) if the collaborative research project she initiated was unsuccessful, or when it ends. It appears that she sees it as an ethical issue to make a success of the collaborative process of the study in order not to reinforce negative perceptions of people with Asperger's.

Why do these challenges occur?

The confidentiality of partners in research and their sensitivity to work carefully with the complex sensitive data is essential. Both academic and community researchers who participate in studies can have privileged positions and do not always foresee the consequences of their work. If they do not reflect on their positions and the risks of participation for people who may be in vulnerable situations, this could enlarge the risks described above.

Dodson and colleagues (2007) relate exploitation to lack of commitment for collaborative meaning-making in the context of contemporary academia, which is focused on production and competition. They note that in positivistic academia 'the interpretive moment in a study is understood as an intellectual province of the scholar, academic or research expert'. Students are trained to find, claim and author originality, explicitly *not* with others. Collaborative work can be regarded as decreasing one's status as researcher in a positivistic research culture.

How can we handle these challenges?

There are no simple signposts on the pathway to handle risks. Risks are very situational. When working together with those whose lives are the subject of the study in the whole process, including analysis and reporting, it is important to assess and discuss risks. This is the basis of protection of people experiencing vulnerability in every stage of the research. Analysis of the data and interpreting together with people whose lives are the subject of the study could be done by Creative Critical Hermeneutic Analysis (van Lieshout & Cardiff, 2011), for example. This is a process of collaborative analysis that brings different voices together and makes sure that voices are heard in analysis.

4) Responsibility for the sustainability of participatory research studies

A quality criterion for participatory research is supporting transformative processes, which go beyond the span of the research study (ICPHR, 2013). In practice, it is possible that resources for participatory research finish and professional researchers leave the setting, before the process of empowerment is completed or the impact of the research is yet visible or achieved (Jamshidi et al., 2014; see also Chapter 7 in this volume). Who is responsible for the sustainability of the outcomes of a research project and who is dependent on whom in these processes?

External funding of participatory research studies places partners in positions of dependence and responsibility (Puffer et al., 2013). What responsibility do initiating partners of participatory research have for obtaining support when the research funding finishes and the project is not implemented sustainably in local structures (Jamshidi et al., 2014; Puffer, 2013)? For what length of time should partners remain actively involved? And how much time and effort are people whose lives are the subject of the study obligated and able to give, particularly if financial compensation decreases or disappears after funding finishes? The difficulty is that people often have little access to potential sources of funding. Other partners could have more easy access to resources, although raising funds could be a full-time job. Jackie Robinson, the academic researcher in Case 2.2, articulates her responsibility to gain funds to continue with the research group of people with Asperger's syndrome.

Why do these challenges occur?

One of the aims of participatory research is transformation through human agency (ICPHR, 2013). Creating positive social change takes often more time and effort than the span of funded research studies. These long-term aims do not fit the 'system' of funding, based on concrete outcomes and short-term planning. Furthermore, activities involving a broad coalition of stakeholders in research and training to carry on the initiatives launched during the research are often not included in funding bids. These activities are not a part of a research project in traditional positivist research. Trust and a shared long-term vision of partners, including funders, is necessary to achieve goals of social transformation.

How can we handle these challenges?

Achieving social transformation by participatory research requires a long time and quick victories are illusory. We can call participatory research 'slow science', a concept borrowed from the 'slow food' movement (Ulmer, 2017). Slow science is a movement formed around the felt need to protect the time of scientists. Adams et al. (2014) describe slow science as a protest against a focus on productivity, multi-tasking, always thinking of the next big thing, scaling up and implementing, often even before we have completed the tasks at hand. This fast approach is often triggered by precarious working conditions. Slow science is 'a response and possible alternative to the newest normative trends' (Adams et al., 2014). It is a different kind of being, requiring a slow ontology (Ulmer, 2017). The plea of slow research is to work more ethically, reciprocally, in more satisfying and helpful ways in an effort to create a better world (Adams et al., 2014; Grandia, 2015). The concept of 'slow research' could help a participatory researcher articulate the need for more time and less rush. A question that could be discussed with partners is: do we together strive towards information acquisition about this subject, or knowledge and social transformation?

PART 2: CASES AND COMMENTARIES

Case 2.1 Power inequities and ethical challenges in action research at public nursing homes in Denmark

Annette Bilfeldt

Introduction

This case is written by an academic researcher and relates to experiences during action research projects undertaken at public nursing homes in Copenhagen, Denmark during 2010–2016. The aim of the projects was to improve the professional skills and engagement of the care workers and to improve the life quality of the residents. The projects followed the core characteristics of action research, focusing on democratic results as well as a democratic process between the participants, who were the manager, employees, residents and academic researchers. The projects were organised with a steering group consisting of representatives from the different participant groups. As a central part of the projects 'future workshops' were employed. This entailed participants collaborating in designing utopias and developing them into plans for new directions for the organisation. These workshops were followed by a conference, where participants presented their solutions in order to fine-tune them with the help of experts and invited guests.

The case

The first project, 'Quality in Eldercare at Nursing Homes from the Staff Perspective', was initiated by the Union for Public Employees and was a joint project between university action researchers and the nursing home. However, the manager of the nursing home did not understand the co-researcher concept. As action researchers we wanted to build up trusting relationships and found the behaviour of the manager disrespectful to employees and residents and to the principle of involvement in the project. Sometimes the manager had 'forgotten' to invite the employees and residents to join the steering group meetings. We felt very unhappy about this situation because we had promised employees and residents that they were a central part of the process during the whole project period. When we asked about the absent members of the steering group, the manager apologised and promised that all the members of the steering group would be invited next time. But it happened several times.

Once when we were going to have a future workshop with the employees at 10 a.m., the manager had ordered the employees to start work at 7 a.m., so they were too tired when they arrived to develop visions and planning during the following five hours. The lack of understanding of the co-researcher concept became even more obvious when the manager suddenly decided to prohibit an employee from taking part in the conference for invited experts. This care worker had played a very important role at the future workshop, because she had interviewed residents about their wishes for social life. Based on the interviews she had developed a utopia about a living room in the centre of the building in order to increase social activities, followed up by a plan for a renovation of the building with 'a town square' in the centre.

When the expert conference was going to be held, the employees who had developed the vision and the plans for the renovation were suddenly ordered to work by the manager instead of joining the conference. The academic researchers tried to convince the manager to change her decision, but we did not succeed. The result of the project was democratic, but the process was not.

In another action research project, 'Improving Life Quality of the Residents and Reducing Stress amongst the Employees', there were examples of employee participants focusing on their own interests at the expense of those of residents and their families. At a future workshop suddenly some of the employees developed what we (academic researchers) regarded as 'dystopias', entailing restrictions that did not address the needs of the residents. A little group of 'hard core' employees started to dominate the development of what should have been visions for the whole nursing home. One vision was about the residents being in bed by 8.30 p.m. in order to enable the evening shift workers to clean the common areas before the night shift arrived. The rationale was to give the night shift a more relaxed night, instead of respecting the residents' interests in keeping autonomy and being able to decide when to go to bed.

Another group developed 'dystopias' which included making a pamphlet for new residents and their relatives about restrictions and rules about life at the nursing homes. This included forbidding bird cages and shelves on the walls in the residents' flats in order to make them easier to clean. My action research colleague and I were not prepared for these dystopias that were in opposition to the aim of improving life quality and autonomy for the residents. And we were in doubt about how to handle the situation. It was clear to us that the other employees did not know how to stop the development of the dystopias, because they were dominated by the little group of "hard core" employees, who were more interested in their own working conditions than in the residents' well-being.

The academic researchers decided to invite the wife of a resident to the expert conference to come and speak about problems she and her husband had faced when he moved into a nursing home. This presentation, which was supported by a broad discussion about being dependent on help from other people, resulted in a new understanding about the importance of the autonomy of residents and their families. Based on that discussion, utopias and plans for more autonomy were developed. The result turned out to be a learning process about the development of a democratic understanding relating to showing respect to the views of the least powerful people at the nursing home. This learning process became an important step in the commencement of a new praxis for involvement of the residents and their relatives in decisions at all levels at the institution.

Reflecting on this case highlights the importance of paying attention to power relations in action research. Action research focuses on democratic results and processes, but as action researchers we have no fixed solutions. The only thing we can do is to be aware of the risk of power inequities and to be ready to handle them when they appear. Nursing homes are work places and homes at the same time. The power of management and employees is stronger than the power of residents and relatives. It is therefore important to reflect on the relations of power and give voice to those who have least power.

Commentary on Case 2.1

Barbara Groot, Melanie Peterman, Ruud van Zuijlen and Tineke Abma

The case seems a realistic example of the complex power dynamics in the context of participatory research, and health care relations in general. Managers and health care workers are motivated to care for and nurture people, but can get caught up in an institutional system that hardly leaves room for the human dimensions. In this case, they seem to find it difficult to both see situations from other people's perspectives, and to work creatively together, even though they share the commitment to care for people. We also recognise situations in which service users are hindered in their autonomy, like the residents in the nursing home. Examples include not being invited to join major decisions, just because service users do not have a position in the hierarchy. Time, trust and a shared long-term vision of partners is necessary to achieve goals of social transformation. Working together, on an equal level of power with service-users, health care workers and managers, seems almost a utopia. As we see in our Community of Practice for Participatory Research, called Centre for Client Experiences, in Amsterdam, it takes time to get somewhere.

If we reflect on this case from a more macro social–economic perspective, we recognise Annette's research as a typical participatory study in times of care reforms and transition. In our practice we also see managers or directors and care workers who resist a redistribution of power. Care and welfare institutions in many countries in Western Europe are transforming from institutions that are organised top-down, internally focussed, without much attention to the autonomy of residents, to institutions in which co-creation and engagement in policy and care of those who live or work in institutions, family, friends and neighbours is high-profile. However, this transformation, which fits the approach of participatory research, is combined with serious budget cuts. More work needs to be done by fewer people (often in flexible, temporary jobs) to realise a higher productivity and efficiency, with a caseload that is heavier, while at the same time demands for improved safety and quality of care increase. No wonder that extra activities are difficult to organise in the face of such precariousness and work pressure. In practice, we see managers and care-workers being very enthusiastic about participatory research, but not open to each other's perspectives because of hierarchical pressure, protocols, and power-lessness in the midst of uncertainty and stress. This broader perspective is our lens to understand the resistance to collaboration in participatory research.

Case 2.2 Participatory research with adults with Asperger's syndrome in the UK

Jackie Robinson

Introduction

This case is written by an academic researcher based in the UK, describing a research project conducted in partnership with people with Asperger's syndrome. It was designed to examine the support needs of people with Asperger's syndrome. Asperger's syndrome is a condition where people experience difficulties with communication with other people as well as understanding social situations. It is considered to be part of the autistic spectrum. In the UK, some local authorities have specific social work teams to support people with Asperger's syndrome, while others use specialist mental health or learning disability teams to give support. Some people with Asperger's syndrome live independently in the community and have successful careers, whereas for others this is a struggle.

The case

The research took place in England between July 2009 and July 2012. It involved myself as a neuro-typical researcher (in this context neuro-typical is someone who does not have autism or Asperger's syndrome) and three co-researchers with

Asperger's syndrome. We conducted the research in partnership, developing every stage of the research together. Together we designed the research tools (a questionnaire and questions for focus groups), conducted focus groups, analysed data and disseminated results at a conference, which we ran ourselves. The aim of the research was to determine what support people with Asperger's syndrome feel they need. We included 30 people with Asperger's syndrome as participants, with some answering questionnaires and others taking part in focus groups. There was an initial questionnaire which participants answered online, or by post, or they requested a one-to-one meeting with the researcher to help complete it. After the data were analysed, two focus groups were held for different participants. The purpose of these was to deepen the understanding of the questionnaire data. The aim was to conduct the research in a participatory way, so my ideas and pre-conceptions as a neuro-typical person would not dominate, but instead would be used to support the co-researchers. I wanted us to ask questions which were relevant to people with Asperger's syndrome and made sense to them. I also wanted to understand the data through the 'lens' of people with Asperger's syndrome. I did not want to impose my way of understanding the data.

I am writing from my point of view as a university researcher. For me, the ethical issues were mainly concerned with how much influence I exerted. I was not aware of any published participatory research with co-researchers with Asperger's syndrome at the time I commenced the research. I wanted to prove that it is possible to have co-researchers with Asperger's syndrome. I wanted to show that it is the way research is conducted that is important and if this is done in an enabling way, then it can be successful. As a social work practitioner, I had attended a lot of training sessions based on a deficit model of understanding Asperger's syndrome. The message I had taken was that people with Asperger's syndrome struggle in all social situations. I had been very influenced by Oliver's (2009) Social Model of Disability in my practice and wanted to explore applying this model to working with people with Asperger's syndrome. I was keen to show that if the environment was not disabling for people, then they would be able to function in a group situation much better. Three main ethical issues arose for me in this project:

1. I wanted to prove a point and felt the weight of that responsibility. If the research was not successful, then I would let the co-researchers down. I had recruited them and would add the research to their list of group situations which had been unsuccessful for them. Fortunately this was not the case, but I did not know this at the beginning.
2. I was concerned about how much I influenced the group. We found a way of working together as a result of me listening to the co-researchers and finding out what they were happy with and what was to be avoided. This worked well and over time we developed a real sense of being a group. We respected what each member was comfortable with. Part of this respect for each other meant that it would have been very easy to have steered the group as the co-researchers listened to me as much as to each other. I did in fact have the role

of keeping the discussions 'on track' as conversations around the data in particular could lead to lengthy discussions about the co-researchers' own experience. I realised quickly that these conversations were very valuable as they shed light on the data and did act as the 'lens' that I was looking for. However, I was often unsure how much steering I should do as I did not want to lose valuable insights, but at the same time I was aware of keeping to the timescales we had agreed.

3. Related to this, I quickly realised what a valuable experience the research was for the co-researchers. They benefitted from the discussions with each other in particular and said that none of them had ever had the opportunity to talk to other adults with Asperger's syndrome about their experiences and what it means to live in a society dominated by neuro-typical people. This presented me with the dilemma of progressing the research, but also allowing the group to have the time to be supportive of each other. This was not difficult to achieve, but required time to be given for the research itself as well as for the valuable support every group member gave to each other. The dilemma I felt very keenly was what were we going to do once the research concluded? All co-researchers were keen to continue to meet up after the research had ended. It was so clear to me that the co-researchers (as well as myself) really benefitted from being a part of our group. Five years after we concluded our research, we are still meeting as a group. I feel a great responsibility to continue what I have started. I look for projects for the group to do so it can continue to work together. So far, we have co-written and published a journal article, been keynote speakers at a conference, taught students at the university where I work and produced a DVD. We are now working on a book.

I have found that taking part in this research has been the greatest challenge of my career, but has also been the most rewarding thing I have ever done. In working in such a participatory way, the co-researchers and I have created a group that has achieved a lot and proved that co-researchers with Asperger's syndrome can be very successful in research. But this has also brought responsibilities. I had read criticisms of non-disabled researchers who just left the co-researchers after the research had ended and used the research to further their own careers. I really did not want to do this and so I have been concerned to continue to support the group. I am aware that I cannot do this with another group, as I do not have the time.

Commentary on Case 2.2

Barbara Groot, Melanie Peterman, Ruud van Zuijlen and Tineke Abma

This case shows us the energy of good collaboration and shared benefits for all involved in a project. This is how we want to collaborate: a good vibe in a group, a shared goal and everybody benefits in a different way. It reminded us that it is important in participatory research to share expectations and perceived benefits of the project among co-researchers in the team. This could generate a feeling of equity and equality. Reserving time to express and talk about everyone's expectations and learning experiences is important. We might do this more often ourselves, because there may be more unexpected benefits than we know. We feel that reflecting on the collaboration can be beneficial.

Often professionals, including researchers, see service users as 'people in need' or 'people that need to be protected'. In this case Jackie was concerned that she should not add to the co-researchers' list of situations that had been unsuccessful. This is a typical dynamic in care, but also in participatory studies between 'disabled' and 'non-disabled' people. People often think 'for' service users, for example people telling a person in a wheelchair it is too far or exhausting to come to a meeting. But why not let people decide for themselves? Professional researchers need to stop thinking for people, and talk to the people concerned.

We have experienced that collaboratively researching each other's responsibility to care in participatory research generated surprising insights. Relationally, it is important to raise the issue of responsibility because this can lead to a new 'sharedness'. If researchers have the courage to show their concerns about responsibility, they show their own vulnerability too. This makes the whole process more shared. From this mutuality all co-researchers may gain strength, and a strong feeling of belonging. This will deepen the partnership, and generate new ideas about what 'partnership' can mean for all.

Case 2.3 Researching gender-based violence in Rwanda: What do we really mean by 'building' local research capacity?

Jenevieve Mannell

Introduction

This case is written by a university-based academic from the UK, who was undertaking research in Rwanda on gender-based violence. Rwanda is a country where 20 per cent of women agree that their husband is justified in beating them if they argue with him, 22 per cent if they go out without telling him, and 24 per cent if they refuse to have sexual intercourse with him (National Institute of Statistics Rwanda, 2016). Gender-based violence against women by husbands/partners is estimated at approximately 40 per cent (Ntaganira et al., 2008).

The case

The majority of my research looks at trying to understand ways to prevent gender-based violence (GBV) in extreme settings, where violence is seen as a normal part of relationships between men and women. For the past five years, I have been working in Rwanda on a project to develop understandings of community responses to GBV and the role played by national gender policies, funded by the London

School of Economics Annual Fund. Within this context, my research team has been conducting interviews with women who have experienced violence, and focus group discussions with community members about strategies for its prevention. A significant focus of this work has been the participation of local researchers as part of an effort to build local research capacity – an objective that is high on the agenda of many international donors. For the project, I specifically recruited two Rwandan women who had previous training in social work from a local university. The purpose of this was to identify women who were recent graduates, would benefit from the additional research skills we could offer and also had some previous training in discussing sensitive topics in order to protect the research participants. I offered these research assistants training in qualitative interviewing and focus group facilitation, and held regular research group discussions before and after interviews/focus groups to discuss any ethical or emotional issues arising from the study. The research assistants were seen as a core part of the research team and were encouraged to ask questions they felt were relevant in addition to the topic guide, reflect on the data being collected, participate in the data analysis, and provide active written input to the published articles and reports. While individuals affected by the issue of GBV in Rwanda were not directly involved in the research process (due to ethical concerns about asking women experiencing violence to interview other women about violence), this approach of involving recent graduates as researchers is consistent with the emphasis in community-based participatory research on systems development and local community capacity building, and a co-learning process where local community members and outside researchers contribute equally.

Despite my best efforts to ensure the full participation of the local researchers, this did not go entirely as planned for reasons I explain in detail. For me, these challenges raise core ethical questions around the meaning of research participation in low-income settings. Data collection went well, and the previous skills and training of the researchers helped to ensure their full participation in this stage of the project. The researchers had their own ideas about what they wanted to explore during the focus groups (e.g. one researcher was interested in dowry and its influence on experiences of gender-based violence), and they were encouraged to do so. However, after data collection was complete it was quite difficult to engage the local researchers in the analysis and writing process. A major part of this was that I could not pay the researchers for their time in this stage of the research. The small grant we received to carry out this piece of work included the direct costs of research activities (e.g. researchers' time in collecting data), and not additional informal collaborative activities (e.g. skype conversations with the research team, or time for writing). This was not a limitation put on us by the funder (although it is often the case that funders place restrictions on the types of research activities they are willing to fund). In our case, the funds available were very small – only £5,000 – and we were therefore only able to cover activities that were absolutely essential for data collection. The local researchers expressed frustration with my efforts to engage them in the analysis and writing process, saying they did not have time to devote to it and preferred to focus on other paid work. Eventually, they stopped responding to emails asking for their input, particularly during the process of writing. One of the local researchers explicitly said she did not want to participate in writing the final articles and would like to be removed as an author from the final papers.

In a context where paid work is largely ad hoc and irregular, this reaction to research participation is hardly surprising. Rwanda is a country undergoing rapid economic development. However a significant proportion of women are either unpaid for the work they do (19 per cent) or are paid through a combination of cash and in-kind (43 per cent) (National Institute of Statistics Rwanda, 2016). There is considerable pressure on young graduates to find work wherever they can, to be multi-skilled and infinitely adaptive. As an academic I value the idea of trying to bring about social change through my research consistent with a community-based participatory research epistemology, however for the local researchers involved in this project, research participation is just another piece of paid work. This makes it extremely challenging to uphold an ideal of participatory research as a political process that involves lay people in theory making. In this case, the ideal of building local capacity runs the risk of becoming a catch-phrase written into funding proposals rather than something that adequately reflects the reality of research on the ground.

Commentary on Case 2.3

Barbara Groot, Melanie Peterman, Ruud van Zuijlen and Tineke Abma

The struggles of the author of this case are recognisable for us, especially because we also work together with all different sorts of people in participatory research, often in academic-led studies, funded externally. We sympathise with the women who do not get paid for their contribution in the analysis and report writing phase. We reflect on our privileged position, living in a Western country in which the government arranges an unemployment benefit if you do not have a job.

Sharing power over resources can be challenging, especially for the initiator. What rights and privileges does an initiator have to allocate resources for (sometimes yet unknown) others and their own activities as a facilitator or academic? To what extent is academic expertise necessary in relation to the shared goals and to the research funder? What is the facilitator's own philosophy about sharing resources at the start and for the long term? What are the needs (for financial compensation) of the people involved in the team? In our experience these questions are all relevant, but there are no easy answers and solutions in practice.

The difficulties are rooted in system logics, expertise and quality standards. Contemporary academic life is precarious. Permanent, fixed positions are rare in universities, leading to insecurity, competition, and an enormous pressure to be academically productive and have social impact (Abma, 2016). So, researchers are expected to raise funds to maintain their own positions at universities. This then implies that both the community-based people involved in the study, as well as the academic researchers, are in precarious positions and in need of resources. This creates tensions in the process of allocation of the budget. Besides, a facilitator needs to have skills and vision, which is essential for the process of participatory research, and frequently participants or people who are the subject of the study may not (yet) be skilled in research. Moreover, the initiator is formally responsible for the quality of the outcome and output of the research for the funder. All these barriers make decisions about sharing resources difficult.

Case 2.4 Starting as you mean to go on: Including young people in a participatory research project in the UK

Candice Satchwell

Introduction

This case was contributed by an academic researcher based in a UK university. It discusses issues arising at the start of a participatory research project with children and young people, regarding how to include them in the interviews for project researchers.

The case

I was Principal Investigator for the first time on a UK research council-funded project entitled 'Stories to Connect', about children's narratives of resilience and transformation. The project, at the University of Central Lancashire (North West England), was a collaboration with the regional unit of Barnardo's, a UK charity supporting vulnerable children. The research team included four academics from different disciplines and myself, supported by the management team at Barnardo's. The university had previously worked with Barnardo's young people aged between 13 and 25 years old through the university's Centre for Children and Young People's Participation. The aim of the new project was to reach out from this group to children and young people with no previous involvement.

At the start we needed to recruit one full-time or two part-time researchers. To fulfil the requirements of our funder and the university, we needed people with PhDs and relevant research experience. However, since the researchers would also be working closely with young people, it was crucial that the young people also regarded them as suitable. The academic team felt we should include young people in the selection process.

However, while we positioned our project as collaborative and participatory (we were working with Barnardo's and training young researchers to work alongside the academic team), ultimately the decision-making power lay with the university. Two academics drew up the short-list of candidates for interview and it would have been easy to go ahead and conduct interviews with only academics on the panel.

However, we decided we should give the young people a say in who would be working with them, and with us.

So, who should the young people be? How would they get to the venue? Would they be able to come on a school day? Who should accompany them? What contribution would they make to the selection process? Could we keep them there all day – there were eight candidates to consider? How much input would they have in the final decision? What if we disagreed? In addition to these questions, when our intention to bring Barnardo's young people into the university became apparent I was also asked, 'Have you done a risk assessment?'

Attempting to establish links with young people willing and able to come on the specified day required liaising with Barnardo's and the County Council. On the day, one Barnardo's worker and one Council worker brought three teenage boys. They had been selected by the workers as young people they had contact with, who were available (two were in care, one was a young carer for his parent, one also had a sight impairment). However, they did not know one another, and first had to establish connections and agreement amongst themselves about how to approach the interviews. They decided on three main activities: an ice-breaker game; a role play involving a bully, a victim and a teacher; and an activity to design a day out for a group of young people with disabilities within a given budget.

To avoid keeping the boys there all day, we allotted two 45-minute sessions for them with four candidates in each. The boys devised a grid system by which to 'grade' the candidates. After the two sessions the boys agreed on their scores, and gave their grid to the three academics on the interview panel (two female project team members and one independent male academic) in a sealed envelope.

At the end of a long day the three academics had to make a decision. The boys, and pretty much everyone else, had gone home. The candidates were a remarkable set of individuals, each with different attributes. Not only did we have to decide whom to appoint, but also whether it was better to have one person or two people, taking into account the preferences expressed by each candidate. As Principal Investigator, I felt the decision was critical for the future of the project. We narrowed our selection down to three or four, but then reached an impasse. At this point we opened the envelope. In retrospect I wonder if we should have opened the envelope sooner – or later? As it happened, the young people's decision helped us. With the young people's feedback we were able finally to settle on one person to fulfil both roles, a candidate that all the academics and all the boys were happy with.

When the boys left us with their envelope, they asked if they could tell the chosen person the good news. Frankly, my heart sank. I wanted that job! And how on earth could it be managed? I didn't have phone numbers for the young people so I would have to go through the workers. I wanted to tell the candidates as soon as possible, and needed to tell the successful one first – what if the boys weren't available at the right time? Which of the boys would it be – it could not be all of them?

As it happened, it could be managed, although not without some effort. I first obtained via their workplaces the mobile phone numbers of the two workers involved; then they contacted the young people for their availability and permission to share their phone numbers with me. The young man who cared for his parent was available but could not leave his house; the others were unavailable. Eventually, after experimenting with my office phone, I arranged a three-way phone call, so that he was able to break the news to our chosen candidate.

Reflecting after the event, our appointed researcher explained how she felt at the end of the interview experience:

> I left feeling dumbfounded by the whole experience and wanted to get the job now more than ever, having had first-hand experience of seeing the young people positioned as real stakeholders of the project and feeling that they seemed to have a real say in major decisions – I was keen to see how this might play out as the project evolved.

The researcher explained to me afterwards her delight in hearing directly from the young man. Her comments about the young people's position as 'real stakeholders' are thought-provoking for us, as the project evolves and we continue to face challenges and dilemmas. Nonetheless, reflecting on the beneficial outcomes of this initial interviewing process leads me to embrace the possibilities of participatory research. It has certainly changed the way I think about the research process, and it will be difficult for me to retreat back to more conventional relationships among participants.

Commentary on Case 2.4

Barbara Groot, Melanie Peterman, Ruud van Zuijlen and Tineke Abma

We are pleasantly surprised about the responsibility the boys received from the academic researchers. We feel this is a very good example from which to learn in relation to our own practice. By inviting the boys to take on the responsible task of working together in the job interview and telling the good news to the chosen young person, the academics shared ownership of the decision-making process. Sharing the responsibility and 'nice jobs' says a lot about how egalitarian people are in relationships.

Besides, this case reminds us about the difficulty of working with participatory research in a traditional organisation with traditional procedures and hierarchical attitudes. It requires flexible thinking and working, as demonstrated by Candice. An example is the question about the risk assessment, which Candice received from her university colleagues. We interpreted this from our own experiences, in which we constantly have to convince people to work differently – especially if you want to share power with people without a title or certificate, like the boys in this case. For us it indicates that people in hierarchical positions of power may fear the loss of power.

If we practise participatory research, one of the principles is to engage those whose lives are the subject of the study in as many phases of the study as possible. In participatory practice it is common to prepare meetings together in a group, meet each other as co-researchers before the start, discuss who wants to be present at meetings and what tasks are available to do. In this case, it seems that the academic researchers decided to involve young people at a rather late stage in the process, which meant that they could not prepare together in advance of the interview day. They also felt that they could not keep the boys and their care workers all day at the university. This meant that the academic researchers had to make the final decision. This raises the question as to whether it could be regarded as patronising and tokenistic, given the age of co-researchers, not to include them in the final decision.

PART 3: CONCLUDING COMMENTS

This chapter shows the importance of reflection on power dynamics, interpersonal relations in micro-contexts, partnerships and collaborations. Participatory research values egalitarian partnerships and mutual caring relationships. These need to be developed and are often under pressure. Collaborative reflections on, and evaluations of, the partnerships are therefore necessary to stay emotionally tuned. This includes exchanging perceptions of responsibility, collaboratively analysing power dynamics and exchanging visions on the macro-economic influences that impact on local collaborations. Such efforts stem from an ethos of 'slow research' (Ulmer, 2017) in order to contribute to social transformation.

References

Abma, T.A. (2016) Tragedy at the modern university, An advocacy for bildung and participatory pedagogy. In: M. Flikkema (Ed.) *Sense of serving, Reconsidering the role of universities now.* (pp. 50–60). VU University Press: Amsterdam.

Abma, T. A., Leyerzapf, H., & Landeweer, E. (2017). Responsive Evaluation in the Interference Zone Between System and Lifeworld. *American Journal of Evaluation, 38*(4), 507–520.

Achkar, J. M., & Macklin, R. (2009). Ethical considerations about reporting research results with potential for further stigmatization of undocumented immigrants. *Clinical infectious diseases, 48*(9), 1250–1253.

Adams, V., Burke, N. J., & Whitmarsh, I. (2014). Slow research: thoughts for a movement in global health. *Medical Anthropology, 33*(3), 179–197.

Bainbridge, R., Tsey, K., Brown, C., McCalman, J., Cadet-James, Y., Margolis, S., & Ypinazar, V. (2013). Coming to an ethics of research practice in a remote Aboriginal Australian community. *Contemporary nurse, 46*(1), 18–27.

Banks, S., Armstrong, A., Carter, K., Graham, H., Hayward, P., Henry, A., . . . & Moore, N. (2013). Everyday ethics in community-based participatory research. *Contemporary Social Science, 8*(3), 263–277.

Boser, S. (2007). Power, ethics, and the IRB dissonance over human participant review of participatory research. *Qualitative Inquiry*, *13*(8), 1060–1074.

Brabeck, K., Lykes, M. B., Sibley, E., & Kene, P. (2015). Ethical ambiguities in participatory action research with unauthorized migrants. *Ethics & Behavior*, *25*(1), 21–36.

Brugge, D., & Kole, A. (2003). A case study of community-based participatory research ethics: the Healthy Public Housing Initiative. *Science and engineering ethics*, *9*(4), 485–501.

Brunger, F., & Wall, D. (2016). 'What Do They Really Mean by Partnerships?' Questioning the Unquestionable Good in Ethics Guidelines Promoting Community Engagement in Indigenous Health Research. *Qualitative health research*, *26*(13), 1862–1877.

Brydon-Miller, M. (2012). Addressing the ethical challenges of community-based research. *Teaching Ethics*, *12*(2), 157–162.

Dodson, L., & Schmalzbauer, L. (2005). Poor mothers and habits of hiding: Participatory methods in poverty research. *Journal of Marriage and Family*, *67*(4), 949–959.

Dodson, L., Piatelli, D. & Schmalzbauer, L. (2007). Researching inequalities through interpretive collaborations: Shifting power and the unspoke contract. *Qualitative Inquiry*, *13*(6), 821–843.

Durham Community Research Team. (2011). *Community-Based Participatory Research: Ethical Challenges*. Durham: Centre for Social Justice and Community Action Durham University, www.ahrc.ac.uk/documents/project-reports-and-reviews/connected-communities/community-based-participatory-research-ethical-challenges/ (accessed January 2018).

Fouché, C. B., & Chubb, L. A. (2017). Action researchers encountering ethical review: a literature synthesis on challenges and strategies. *Educational Action Research*, *25*(1), 23–34.

Grandia, L. (2015). Slow ethnography: A hut with a view. *Critique of Anthropology*, *35*(3), 301–317.

Graham, J. W. (1991). Servant-leadership in organizations: Inspirational and moral. *The Leadership Quarterly*, *2*(2), 105–119.

Greenleaf, R.K. (1977) *Servant leadership*. New York: Paulist Press.

Habermas, J. (1987). *The Philosophical Discourse of Modernity*. Cambridge: Polity Press.

International Collaboration for Participatory Health Research (ICPHR) (2013). *Position Paper 1: What is Participatory Health Research?* Version: May 2013. Berlin: International Collaboration for Participatory Health Research.

Jamshidi, E., Morasae, E. K., Shahandeh, K., Majdzadeh, R., Seydali, E., Aramesh, K., & Abknar, N. L. (2014). Ethical considerations of community-based participatory research: Contextual underpinnings for developing countries. *International Journal of Preventive Medicine*, *5*(10), 1328.

Janes, J. E. (2016). Democratic encounters? Epistemic privilege, power, and community-based participatory action research. *Action Research*, *14*(1), 72–87.

Kemmis, S. (2008). Critical theory and participatory action research. In P. Reason and H. Bradbury (Eds.), *The SAGE handbook of action research: Participative inquiry and practice*, 2nd edn (pp. 121–138). Thousand Oaks, Calif: SAGE.

Kemmis, S., & McTaggart, R. (2005). Communicative action and the public sphere. In N.K. Denzin & Y.S. Lincoln (Eds.), *The SAGE handbook of qualitative research*, 3rd edn (pp. 559–603). Thousand Oaks, Calif: SAGE.

Kuriloff, P. J., Andrus, S. H., & Ravitch, S. M. (2011). Messy ethics: conducting moral participatory action research in the crucible of university–school relations. *Mind, Brain, and Education*, *5*(2), 49–62.

Letiecq, B., & Schmalzbauer, L. (2012). Community-based participatory research with Mexican migrants in a new rural destination: A good fit? *Action Research*, *10*(3), 244–259.

Lincoln, Y. (2009). Ethical practices in qualitative research. In D. M. Mertens & P. E. Ginsberg (Eds.), *The handbook of social research ethics* (pp. 150–169). Thousand Oaks, CA: SAGE.

Love, K. (2011) Little known but powerful approach to applied research: Community-based participatory research. *Geriatric Nursing, 32*(1), 52–54.

Mertens, D. M. (2008). *Transformative research and evaluation.* New York: The Guilford Press.

Mertens, D. M., & Ginsberg, P. E. (2008). Deep in ethical waters: Transformative perspectives for qualitative social work research. *Qualitative Social Work, 7*(4), 484–503.

Mikesell, L., Bromley, E., & Khodyakov, D. (2013). Ethical community-engaged research: a literature review. *American Journal of Public Health, 103*(12), e7–e14.

Minkler, M. (2004). Ethical challenges for the 'outside' researcher in community-based participatory research. *Health Education & Behavior, 31*(6), 684–697.

National Institute of Statistics Rwanda. (2012). *Demographic and Health Survey 2010 – Final Report.* Kigali, Rwanda: Ministry of Finance and Economic Planning. Retrieved from www.statistics.gov.rw/publications/demographic-and-health-survey-2010-final-report (accessed January 2018).

National Institute of Statistics Rwanda. (2016). *Demographic and Health Survey 2014/2015 – Key findings.* Kigali, Rwanda: Ministry of Finance and Economic Planning, www.statistics.gov.rw/publication/demographic-and-health-survey-dhs-20142015-key-findings (accessed January 2018).

Ntaganira, J., Muula, A. S., Masaisa, F., Dusabeyezu, F., Siziya, S., & Rudatsikira, E. (2008). Intimate partner violence among pregnant women in Rwanda. *BMC Women's Health, 8*(1), 17. http://doi.org/10.1186/1472-6874-8-17

O'Neill, C., Harding, A., Harper, B., Stone, D., Berger, P., Harris, S., & Donatuto, J. (2012). Conducting Research with Tribal Communities: Sovereignty, Ethics, and Data-Sharing Issues. *Environmental Health Perspectives, 120*(1), 6–10.

Ochocka, J., Janzen, R., & Nelson, G. (2002). Sharing power and knowledge: professional and mental health consumer/survivor researchers working together in a participatory action research project. *Psychiatric Rehabilitation Journal, 25*(4), 39–58.

Oliver, M. (2009) *Understanding the Social Model of Disability: From Theory to Practice.* Basingstoke: Palgrave Macmillan.

Puffer, E. S., Pian, J., Sikkema, K. J., Ogwang-Odhiambo, R. A., & Broverman, S. A. (2013). Developing a family-based HIV prevention intervention in rural Kenya: challenges in conducting community-based participatory research. *Journal of Empirical Research on Human Research Ethics, 8*(2), 119–128.

Reason, P., & Torbert, W. (2001). The action turn: Toward a transformational social science. *Concepts and Transformation, 6*(1), 1–37.

Rooke, D., & Torbert, W. R. (2005). Seven transformations of leadership. *Harvard Business Review, 83*(4), 66–76.

Salmon, A., Browne, A. J., & Pederson, A. (2010). 'Now we call it research': participatory health research involving marginalized women who use drugs. *Nursing Inquiry, 17*(4), 336–345.

Shore, N. (2006). Re-conceptualizing the Belmont Report: A community-based participatory research perspective. *Journal of Community Practice, 14*(4), 5–26.

Smith, E., Ross, F., Donovan, S., Manthorpe, J., Brearley, S., Sitzia, J., & Beresford, P. (2008). Service user involvement in nursing, midwifery and health visiting research: a review of evidence and practice. *International Journal of Nursing Studies, 45*(2), 298–315.

Souleymanov, R., Kuzmanović, D., Marshall, Z., Scheim, A. I., Mikiki, M., Worthington,

C., & Millson, M. P. (2016). The ethics of community-based research with people who use drugs: results of a scoping review. *BMC Medical Ethics*, *17*(1), 25.

Torbert, W.R. (2003) *Personal and organizational transformations through action inquiry*. London: The Cromwell Press.

Torbert, W. R. (2004). *Action inquiry: The secret of timely and transforming leadership*. San Francisco, CA: Berrett-Koehler Publishers.

Ulmer, J. B. (2017). Writing slow ontology. *Qualitative Inquiry*, *23*(3), 201–211.

Van Dierendonck, D. (2011). Servant leadership: A review and synthesis. *Journal of management*, *37*(4), 1228–1261.

Van Lieshout, F., & Cardiff, S. (2011). Innovative Ways of Analysing Data With Practitioners as Co-Researchers. In J. Higgs, A. Titchen, D. Horsfall & D. Bridges (Eds.) *Creative Spaces for Qualitative Researching* (pp. 223–234). Rotterdam: Sense Publishers.

Walsh, C. A., Hewson, J., & Shier, M. (2008). Unraveling ethics: Reflections from a community-based participatory research project with youth. *The Qualitative Report*, *13*(3), 379–393.

Wilson, E., Kenny, A., & Dickson-Swift, V. (2018). Ethical Challenges in Community-Based Participatory research: A Scoping Review. *Qualitative Health Research*, *28*(2), 189–199.

3

BLURRING THE BOUNDARIES BETWEEN RESEARCHER AND RESEARCHED, ACADEMIC AND ACTIVIST

Anne MacFarlane and Brenda Roche

With cases contributed by Pinky Shabangu, Catherine Wilkinson, Mieke Cardol and Geralyn Hynes

PART 1: INTRODUCTION AND OVERVIEW OF THE ISSUES

Anne MacFarlane and Brenda Roche

Co-production of research for action: implications for the roles and identities for stakeholders

Theoretical underpinnings of participatory research (PR) emphasise some degree of co-production of research and an action orientation. The co-production of knowledge is underpinned by values about equality of knowledges, meaning that there is a particular interest in ensuring that *insider* or *emic* knowledge held within communities is acknowledged, respected and made explicit in the research process. The intended outcome is to produce an authentic and comprehensive account of problems/issues from all perspectives and, with that, appropriate solutions to bring about concrete actions and change.

The emphasis in PR on co-production of research and action orientation has many implications. This chapter is about implications for the roles and identities for the stakeholders involved in PR with a focus on the ways in which *boundaries are blurred*. For example, the emphasis on co-production of knowledge can lead to new roles for community members and professional researchers that layer on top of their existing ones.

Community members may take on researcher roles to bring knowledge to, and from, their community in relation to the research process. Professional researchers may take on roles commonly associated with community development or community action work such as lobbying for health service or policy change. Practitioner researchers may have to consider how their identities as researchers layer on top of their therapeutic identities. Sometimes, these new identities can blur the 'original' ones. For example, community partners may find themselves navigating new layers of their identities in relationships with their peers as a function of their commitment to co-production of knowledge. No longer quite full peers in their communities, or no longer 'only' full peers in their communities, they are privy to new insights and knowledge about problems being explored and methods of inquiry. For professional researchers there are changes too, as they develop relationships with community members as colleagues, and community members then are no longer viewed as participants or aides in research.

Furthermore, and this is a central theme in this chapter, for all parties involved in participatory research the co-production of knowledge hinges on *relationality*. Community members who work as researchers come with an experiential understanding of the community and a range of personal relationships, which can translate into ways to support access or 'reach' to participants for research. Through the very process of co-production, academic researchers and community researchers work together as colleagues, which relies on the active building of relationships between them. In this way, the centrality of the relational in PR means that the boundaries between community and academic spaces, between personal and professional spaces and between formal and informal interactions may become more blurred, and less defined.

This is different from other kinds of research and partnerships between academics and community organisations where there is collaboration for more instrumental purposes, for example, support from a community organisation at the point of recruitment only to administer a questionnaire designed by academics. These differences are the *strengths* of participatory research. However, they can also raise unexpected challenges and ethical complications. In this chapter, we discuss some of these. After a broad overview of literature about ethics and community research, we will focus on three, interconnected, themes. The first is about the *integrity of research methods* when co-producing knowledge. We explore what can happen when academic and community sources of knowledge are blended, and how this may fuel 'clashes' with notions of rigour in research procedures. The second theme centres on *social relationships*, focusing particularly on community researchers and the tensions that can arise as they inhabit two worlds of 'academia' and 'community' at the same time. The third is about *points of action and change* in participatory research. We examine tensions that can arise when desired changes do not occur and consider impacts for the relationships. Finally, we also consider the unanticipated, 'ripple effects' and some of the ethical dilemmas that they pose.

We explore these themes from our perspectives as social scientists. We have backgrounds in psychology, sociology and health promotion (MacFarlane) and anthropology and public health (Roche). In our work we have both developed research programmes which prioritise participation and have worked in close partnership with community-based NGOs and health sector stakeholders, as well as policy-makers. We have seen how the values and principles of participatory research are enacted in real space and time. Through this, and, in the process, we have witnessed the blurring of boundaries in participatory research many times. This has left us with both a sense of *appreciation* about the complexity and richness of this way of researching but, also, some *concerns* about ethical issues. For example, we have seen the benefits of co-researching on recruitment, the development of research instruments and interpretation of research findings. But, also, we have seen how co-researchers have had to grapple with transitions in their role(s) within communities and challenging or shifting dynamics in their social networks. We have struggled with our own roles and the boundaries between academic and activist or advocate. These very divergent roles may come with distinctive understandings of the work itself: how it is practised and what are its outcomes. What amount of time and effort should we, as academics, spend mixing with policy-makers and politicians to 'champion' the findings of participatory projects? And, how do these relationships alter the intent and the nature of the work itself: do they blur the boundaries of the work? It is from this perspective, and with these critical discussions and debates in mind, that we reflect on the literature and, also, comment on four case examples.

Case 3.1 is about a community researcher in Southern Africa who describes the tensions of administering a health survey that involved asking questions of people she knew. This explores how 'insider' knowledge clashed with the integrity of research methods as the community researcher had personal knowledge about a survey participant (who was also a neighbour) that made stringent or exacting adherence to the survey protocol problematic. Was it more ethical to stick rigidly to the protocol or to adjust it to interact sensitively with the person involved?

Case 3.2 is based on doctoral research in England which had a participatory design and, also, involved ethnographic participant observation. The project focused on collaboration with young people at a radio station to understand social capital. The academic researcher reflects on blurred boundaries between researcher and friend as she built up close relationships with some of the young people involved. She had to consider the ethical implications of how that impacted on information shared informally by one young person about their mental health. Was this information being shared with her as a researcher or a friend and what were the implications for its use in the PhD?

Case 3.3, from a university researcher in the Netherlands, continues the theme about researcher versus friend. The case is based on a research project with and about people with intellectual disabilities. Ethical dilemmas surface as the community researchers and academic researchers establish a collegial relationship over time. This growing relationship enhances the reflective process about their lives as well as the research itself. What is 'off the record' and what is data becomes increasingly unclear, as information is obtained informally as a function of close and trusting relationships.

Finally, Case 3.4 is from an academic in Ireland who worked with nurses and an artist to design a PhotoVoice project to open conversations among health care professionals and patients about illness experiences. This moves our attention to ethical dilemmas that arise because of the blurred boundaries that surround the use of innovative research methods for data generation and analysis. The insights that emerge through arts-informed methods may bear a close resemblance to therapeutic processes that rely on reflexive strategies to effect change. How can such unanticipated, 'ripple effects', mentioned earlier, be regarded and responded to?

Ethics and community research

The nature of the participatory research paradigm – regardless of the specific participatory tradition or methodology underscoring the work – raises unique ethical tensions and challenges for community and academic partners engaged in the work. The core characteristics that underpin the participatory research paradigm include a commitment to inclusion in research, where partners work collectively to share their respective knowledges and to pursue and conduct research that is locally situated, and aims to create transformation and action. These have been strongly embraced within Participatory Health Research (see International Collaboration on Participatory Health Research [ICPHR], 2013).

Central to participatory approaches is an understanding of community members and their representatives *working alongside* academic researchers to address and resolve real-world dilemmas and issues. In the literature, community researchers have come to represent individuals with lived experience of issues, reflecting the perspective of community members as colleagues in research or as peer researchers working on research studies (Warr et al., 2012). Researchers are encouraged to think about knowledge transfer and implementation of findings as much as the methodological rigour behind data generation and analysis (Goodson and Phillimore, 2012; ICPHR 2013)

These very characteristics of participatory research, which make it unique and offer value then, are the same elements that can give rise to ethical concerns and tensions: the cardinal dimensions of participatory research, the spaces where it is conducted, and the research encounter itself. These all surface key issues and opportunities that warrant attention. In particular, they raise questions about how the lines between research, action and collective inquiry intersect and where there is potential for a blurring of roles and boundaries.

While ethical review committees focus on contractual ethics, relating to the operational aspects of community research (e.g. processes for data protection and ensuring confidentiality for research participants who complete surveys, interviews and so on: see Brydon Miller, 2009), they cannot identify all the possible issues that can surface for, and between, the academic and community partners working alongside each other, particularly in terms of relationships and roles (McLaughlin 2005). The relational aspects of the work can be difficult to anticipate.

Yet, these issues are critical to the work. Kothari (2001) argues that the material practices, that is the tools and techniques that are used to enact partnership, can shape the nature and quality of partnership. Certainly, there are valuable resources in the PR literature about these and how they may be used to create the space (physically and relationally) to foster meaningful and democratic interactions that emphasise equal status and participation in decision making and research governance (see examples of Participatory Learning and Action research resources in Chambers, 2002; O'Reilly-de Brún et al., 2017).

While there is a body of work about community researchers in participatory research projects, it is striking that in much health and social research literature there is an absence of open recognition of *dilemmas* that can arise for community and academic researchers alike. Much of what is written emphasises the strengths of involving community members in research, not the tensions or uncertainties that may arise in the process (Mosavel and Sanders, 2014). Yet, it is here, within the 'everyday ethics' (Banks et al., 2013) of participatory research that the fundamental nature of participatory research emerges and critical insights for extending knowledge and practice will emerge.

Covenantal ethics provides a good framework for understanding these issues (see Chapter 1 in this volume). Covenantal ethics draws attention to the centrality of participation in participatory research and it offers a different perspective to the contractual ethics focus of research ethics committees mentioned above. Covenantal ethics is an 'ethical stance enacted through relationship and commitment to working for the good of others' that is an inherent component of action research (Brydon Miller, 2009: 244). This stance links with feminist approaches to ethics such as the ethics of care (see Chapter 1 in this volume, pages 11-13) and guidelines developed to support work with indigenous and minority communities, such as the Canadian Institute of Health Research Guidelines for Health Research with Aboriginal Communities (CIHR, 2007). It is about shifting attention to the nature of the ethical issues that arise as the core values of participatory research are enacted and, of course, what responses are required.

The nature of roles in projects, and notions of the boundaries that exist between them, are seldom intentionally set out at the outset of a project. Usually discussions of roles focus more intently on the tasks of research. It is in the enacting of research that the relational comes to life, and the balancing of competing roles and interests become more apparent. What tensions arise as the complexity of relationships unfold, given the multiple and intersecting roles that different stakeholders have as they come together to co-produce knowledge? What tensions arise for individuals because of crossing boundaries between different identities or when trying to interact and broker different ways of seeing and doing things across boundaries of different spaces? Furthermore, who knows or decides when a boundary has been crossed or challenged in some way? The idea of 'boundary-spanners' and 'boundary-crossers' found in Wenger's work on communities of practice is very relevant to academic and community partnerships, as outlined by Hart and Aumann (2012) and to the ethics of conducting PR.

Ethical challenges related to the integrity of research methods when co-producing knowledge

Looking at the recent literature, there is a growing sense that tensions can emerge as community researchers navigate between their understanding of what is appropriate from a community perspective, and what is vital to ensure the integrity of research methods in practice (Flicker et al., 2010; Richman et al., 2015). Likewise, for academic researchers, the balance between the interests of working collaboratively and valuing relationship development with communities may strain against perceptions of maintaining methodological objectivity and rigour.

The ambiguities in relationships can amplify the intense and emotional nature of PR for researchers as they work across social locations (Mosavel et al., 2011). For community researchers, this can be especially profound, where they face unique challenges balancing a new role that is simultaneously a community insider and outsider (Greene et al., 2009). Richman et al., (2012; 2015) build on these ideas, noting that for community researchers their position between community and academic worlds can create a blurring between roles. For some this can play out as a disconnect between what they do in practice and what are the tasks specific to their roles as community researchers. In Case 3.1, this dilemma arises when a community researcher is privy to personal information about a participant, by virtue of being an insider from the community of interest. This poses challenges when faced with administering a research survey.

Cases 3.2 and 3.3 illustrate tensions at the boundaries of the professional relationship between academic and community researchers, bringing our attention to the question of friendship: where does the research partnership begin and end? This is critical to understanding what the relationship looks like, but, also, to the question of what are the limits to data collection where information is shared that is 'off the record'. In relationships between members of a research team, whether as friends or as colleagues, there are points of interaction that may be about establishing or maintaining the relationship itself through personal stories or shared insights rather than intending to add to, or strengthen, the data. How these points of contact are understood by team members however, may differ, reflecting more ambiguous understandings of their relationships with one another.

The negotiation of such roles and personal values is complicated for community and academic researchers alike. However, as Richman and colleagues argue, the *proximity* of community researchers to the community of interest can intensify these issues. Greene (2013) writes of a situation which resonates strongly with Case 3.1: a peer researcher when part-way through an interview, realises that she knows the interviewee's partner. In that moment, she realises that she knows information of which the participant is unaware. Here the peer researcher is between two worlds: she is balancing the competing interests of maintaining confidentiality as a researcher, and acting in the interests of the interviewee as a member of her community. The challenge is how to balance the rules of research, against instincts that are shaped by a sense of commitment to the social relationships that form part of her community.

Ethical challenges for community researchers and their social relationships

Flicker and colleagues (2010) also raise the point that when community researchers are in close proximity to the community of interest, it may foster situations where they are recruiting or collecting data as peers on members of their social circle. They note one situation where a peer researcher on a study acknowledged their commitment to minimising attrition on a research study meant that they compromised their own safety – opting to stay in an abusive relationship rather than jeopardise the data collection. Such a scenario may be rare, but it speaks to how the action of the work can become tied to individual experiences of accomplishment – and the risks or compromises that people may take.

For others, while less hazardous, their position in relation to the community of interest can create unique challenges as they seek to enable or assist local participants through research (True et al., 2011). This new-found position can place them in uneasy roles vis-à-vis other community members. For example, one of us (MacFarlane) was involved in a PR project in Ireland designed to improve communication between asylum seekers and refugees and their general practitioners. Members of the asylum-seeking and refugee community were trained as peer researchers (see MacFarlane et al., 2009). The project included regional health service colleagues and findings and recommendations were included in a subsequent National Intercultural Health Strategy (2007–2012) thus providing some satisfaction around action orientation. However, changes in clinical settings did not follow from the evidence-based strategy. A subsequent evaluation with the peer researchers revealed that, while they were overwhelmingly positive about their experience in the research, there were some unintended consequences. They explained that after the research ended, they often bumped into people from their community in the supermarket, at schools and so on, who had participated in the fieldwork. They were often asked 'What happened with that research?" People wanted to know why the identified solution (provision of trained interpreters) had not been achieved. The implementation of trained interpreters in general practice settings is, however, a tremendously complex translational gap (Greenhalgh et al., 2007; van den Muisjenbergh et al., 2014). Essentially, because of their 'insider' status and as enablers of the fieldwork, the peer researchers had become the 'face' of the research. This meant that they had inadvertently ended up carrying some responsibility for changes in practice that were simply not within their control. These unintended consequences compounded the tensions felt by MacFarlane, as the academic lead, that the research had failed to change practice. This disappointment was all the more keenly felt given the nature of the relationships that had been built up with the peer researchers. Furthermore, it highlighted tensions between academic and activist roles for team members: could or should the academic have done more to ensure findings shaped policy *and* practice? Did the lack of impact on practice, which would have transformed access to health care for the community involved, compromise its inherent ethical and political engagement to achieve social change (Brydon-Miller, 2009)?

This raises the intent of participatory research, where research is the vehicle for social change and transformation, but it should be also read as raising questions about the boundaries of how community researchers work with their communities, and where points of action or change are located.

Ethical challenges regarding points of action and change in participatory research

For community researchers, there can be a willingness to go above and beyond the scope of a researcher role to assist community participants in some way. This can take the shape of offering personal support and ongoing contact outside of the research context to engaging in the 'invisible work' that has been noted in participatory research: where academic researchers offer instrumental assistance that can include escorting community researchers to appointments, and accessing resources (Roche, 2008; Roche, Guta, & Flicker 2010). Case 3.4 provides an example of how this takes shape for an academic researcher who must consider the competing goals of the research encounter versus the therapeutic relationship. Here the lines between research and therapy blur, for example, when a research technique (PhotoVoice) is used to explore illness experiences with patients and yields insights suggestive of a therapeutic intervention. While not intended to serve as therapeutic, the reflexive process that is critical to participatory research (particularly arts-based research) can unintentionally produce important insights for individuals as they reflect on their experiences of health and well-being.

Therefore, overall, we can see that the fluidity of how methods, actions, and interactions operate on a PR project can yield nuanced insights and important results. At the same time, there is ambiguity for all involved as they straddle the roles of community member, researcher and research participant. Increasingly for community and academic researchers alike there are also competing interests as practitioners, advocates and decision-makers within health and social care systems. These can play out in ways that may raise similar questions about the nature of their identities on projects, and the boundaries of their roles and relationships as they struggle to balance or meet what can be competing interests at once. The case studies in the next section of this chapter offer critical insights into these issues.

PART 2: CASES AND COMMENTARIES

Case 3.1 Following research protocols versus being sensitive to informants' feelings: Ethical issues for a community researcher in Southern Africa

Pinky Shabangu

Introduction

This case example is contributed by a community researcher who was undertaking a health survey that involved asking questions of people she knew. In scientific survey research, data collectors are expected to ask exactly the same questions to all participants, to ensure the data is good quality (an important ethical issue, there is no point wasting participants' time if the data collected is not good quality). However, answering some questions can be painful for participants (e.g. if they need to talk about death of a close family member) and that can make it hard for data collectors to ask. This may be particularly so in participatory research, because data collectors often know the participants of whom they ask questions, and may also 'know' the answers to some of the questions they are asking, as was the experience in this case.

The case

The participatory health research I took part in was in my community, a rural southern African community with a population of about 1000. It is in a mountainous area, in a country that has amongst the highest HIV prevalence in the world. It is a small community where everyone knows each other and what is going on in other people's lives (e.g. we attend funerals when somebody in the community has died).

We started the research when a White woman (I will call her Jane) from a developed country, who had been working on community development projects with women in my community for about five years, wanted to do a study of our community for her university degree. She asked for people who wanted to work as researchers on the project to apply, and I did, because I wanted to have a go, as it was something I had never done before. There was no need for previous related experience, the only requirement was to be able to read and write in English.

We (myself and seven other community members) started our jobs as researchers by having a series of training workshops – we learnt about research and ethics and designed a survey and other tools for the project. Then we started collecting the data.

One day Jane came with me, to observe while I was collecting survey data at homesteads in the community. At the first homestead we visited, a young man was the respondent. He was about my age and we had attended primary school together and lived in the same community all our lives. The first section of the questionnaire included demographic questions like age and sex, for each member of the households. For children, we asked whether or not their mother and father were alive or dead. I knew that the respondent's mother had died after being very ill for quite a long time, about a year earlier. Knowing about his mother's death and having to ask this question, I felt it might be offensive to the respondent and I felt a bit foolish asking a question I already 'knew' the answer to. But I felt like I had to ask, because that is what I had been taught to do in the workshops (I was not supposed to assume I knew the answers).

I asked the demographic questions about his first sibling, and when I asked whether or not the siblings' mother was dead, he replied, 'obvious' (in English – we were otherwise communicating in our mother tongue). That is when I began to think that if I continued asking the same question, to which he had already indicated the answer was 'obvious', that I would hurt the participant more because the question dealt with an issue that was sensitive to him. If it was not a sensitive question, for example, if it was about water or farming, I might have just explained that I wanted to hear the answer from him, even though it was 'obvious'. I'm quite sure that if I was not with Jane, instead of saying 'obvious' he would have said something more direct like, 'Are out of your mind to ask me about that?'

I continued with the survey and asked most of the demographic questions for his other sibling, but when I got to the question about their mother being dead, I did not ask, I just recorded the answer. I knew that the mother was dead. I could not bring myself to ask the painful question I already know the answer to again. I felt very uncomfortable asking about his dead mother because I knew that when I asked again he would feel pain. He had already said it was obvious. At that moment, I didn't even think about breaking the data collection rules, I just did it. It was only later when Jane discussed it with me, that I realised this was not how I had been taught to collect the data – I was supposed to record what the respondent told me, not what I thought was the right answer.

But even knowing this, I was not sure if I had done the right thing, or the wrong thing. Would it have been more ethical to cause the participant pain by asking again just to follow the rules (and potentially get better quality data)? In the training, we had not discussed about what to do when you come up with such a situation. I did what I thought was right for the participant and what I felt comfortable doing. I could just imagine if I kept on asking the participant about his dead mother and he started crying. I did not want to keep on reminding the participant about her death.

Commentary on Case 3.1

Anne MacFarlane and Brenda Roche

In PR, community members may take on the role of peer researchers to bring knowledge to, and from, their community in relation to the research process. This is a significant embodiment of the co-production of knowledge. It respects and, in fact, relies on the 'insider' status that community members have. It also highlights the relationships *within* community, between community members. It draws our attention to the role of peer researchers as a bridge between the community and the academy (O'Reilly-de Brún et al., 2016).

In this case, the community researcher makes a judgement call to 'deviate' from the research protocol to honour the personal knowledge she held as a function of her status as 'insider'. This reminds us that while the relational nature of PR is its strength, and that working with peer researchers can be so valuable for the academy, we cannot assume that it is always positive, easy or free from ethical dilemmas for those who take on the new identity as 'researcher'. Like other identities, the new identity of researcher is fluid and when the PR project has ended, the identity of peer researcher may fade but the identity as a community member will not. In this instance, strict adherence to study protocols for methodological rigour would, arguably, have been insensitive to the survey participant and have perhaps 'diminished' the personal relationship between him and the peer researcher. This case shows the importance of debriefing during fieldwork. This is a key action in PR processes. It allows unanticipated dilemmas like this to be named, recorded and reflected upon in a supportive manner. The nuances of when, in fact, it is an ethical action for community researchers to amend an agreed protocol can be explored and shared with others.

Case 3.2 Are you telling me this as a researcher or a friend? Ethical issues for a UK doctoral researcher

Catherine Wilkinson

Introduction

This case is based on the experiences of a doctoral student undertaking research in Knowsley in the UK. The PhD was exploring how and to what extent a *volunteer youth-led community radio station* provides a space for young people to find and realise their voices.

The case

This case draws on fieldwork for my doctoral research, conducted between March 2012 and September 2015. The main objectives of this study were to:

1. Explore the notion of 'youth voice' in relation to a youth-led radio station.
2. Develop understandings of community in relation to a community radio station, for listeners, staff and volunteers.
3. Establish the ways in which the radio station enhances both 'bonding' social capital (within particular communities) and 'bridging' social capital (across social divides and groups) for both listeners and volunteers.
4. Develop a participatory approach to documenting the value of a community radio station.

This research project adopted a participatory design in collaboration with young people at the radio station. Mixed methods were employed, including: 18 months of participant observation; interviews and focus groups with volunteers; interviews with management; a listener survey, listener diaries, and follow-up interviews. I trained the young people as co-researchers, leading to their involvement in designing and refining interview questions for management through mind-mapping sessions, assisting in data gathering through peer-led focus groups, co-producing the listener survey and assisting with data collection through distributing this survey. Accompanying my thesis were two co-produced audio artefacts: an audio documentary, 'Community to me is . . .', exploring young people's understandings of community; and a three-part radio series, 'What we found', in which the young people discussed the research findings. The young people assisted in recording and editing these audio artefacts, and chose the music clips to be included. I intended my role in the production of these audio artefacts to be that of facilitator, but some young people were reluctant to take on editing, so I assisted with this. The role of the young people as both co-researchers and research informants added complexity in terms of demarcating clear expectations for participation. Despite participating at various stages of the research, including the audio dissemination, I did not invite the young people to participate in writing, due to pressures to submit my PhD thesis within three years.

I visited the radio station four or five days a week, between 08.00 and 20.00 for 18 months. During this time, I formed friendships with many young volunteers and staff members. I did not desire the young people to perceive me as the 'omnipotent expert', so I positioned myself as 'researcher as friend'. This, to me, felt natural as I was similar in age to many of the young people. I believed this gave me an advantage in building rapport, which could lead to strengthened trust and, therefore, greater access to data. Some examples of how I built this friendship include: I accepted the young people's 'friend requests' on Facebook; I passed on my mobile phone number; I invited volunteers to call me by my nickname; and I enjoyed activities with the young people outside of the station, including cinema excursions, shopping sprees and celebratory meals.

At the time of writing my methodology as part of my PhD thesis, and reflecting on researcher positionality, I found it problematic that academic writing believes that you can only be a 'researcher' or a 'friend', but not both. I believed that I could be a genuine friend to the young people and, as such, I sought to create a relationship based on mutual respect. Of course, it must be emphasised that this friendship was in line with their awareness that I was collecting data. My research project was staggered with different activities (e.g. interviews, follow-up interviews, focus groups, listener survey, and the co-production of audio artefacts). I found this useful for reminding young people of my role, both formally (through acts that required participants, for instance, to read information sheets and to sign consent forms), and informally through acts that were associated with research and thus implied my role as a researcher.

Also useful was a poster produced by station management of 'key members' at the radio station. My photograph was on this poster and a description of me as a 'PhD researcher'. The poster was placed prominently on a wall of the station, and remained there throughout my research. Further, my role as a researcher was reaffirmed through a presenter biography on the station website. However, I did not consider these more passive acts, which required the young people to see this information, to be enough. Other, more active, strategies included emphasising my role as a researcher through conversations. For instance, I informed young people of academic conferences I was attending and publications I was writing, as reminders of my role. Thus, whilst young people told me things which they were aware would end up in my thesis, and resultant publications, I told young people things that I was aware would end up used as on-air content. We each had our own duties at the station, but this did not deny our friendships.

One day a young volunteer pulled up a seat next to me, and as if out of nowhere started telling me about his past battles with depression and drug abuse, and how the station had been his saviour. 'What excellent data!' I thought. However, alarm bells rang in my mind, and I asked the young person: 'Are you telling me this as a researcher or a friend?' 'As a friend,' he replied, 'but you can use it in your thesis if you want.' I suddenly began to question my entire approach to this participatory research project, which had drawn me into friendships with young people, which I considered to be inevitable due to our comparable age, our liking of the same music, and our mutual interest in radio. I was left asking myself a series of questions: Is it ethical to build friendships with research participants? Would it be equally unethical to deny research participants' friendship? To what extent can informal discussions, which are an essential part of ethnographic research, be considered ethically sound for inclusion in written reports of our findings? How could I guarantee that other participants had not told me stories as a friend, rather than as a researcher?

In attempting to right any potential wrongs, I sent all young people transcripts of their interviews, and any field notes I had written containing excerpts of their speech. I asked them to let me know if there were any sections of the transcripts they would like me to remove. All young people approved transcripts with no changes. Again, I was left thinking: have they approved the transcripts because I am their friend? But equally, I questioned whether they would be more likely to tell me that they were unhappy with something as their friend, as opposed to a 'big scary researcher'.

Commentary on Case 3.2

Anne MacFarlane and Brenda Roche

In Case 3.2 we encounter one of the unintended effects of academic and community partners working closely together. Here, the lead researcher (PhD student) acknowledges the distinctions that exist between herself and the peer researchers on the study. However, there is a boundary issue as the relationship between the student and the young people is complicated by notions of friendship. It is also complicated by the fact that although there is an element of peer research in the project, the overall design and implementation of the research are the responsibility of the PhD student. The student is also undertaking an ethnographic study, involving participant observation, interviews and focus groups – meaning that the young people are at different times both research informants and co-researchers. This creates another boundary issue for the doctoral researcher of 'ethnographer vs co-researcher', which can be common in participatory research.

The lead researcher in this case focuses on the 'researcher versus friend', boundary. It is not unusual for research partners to develop friendships during the research process itself. However, it is critical to remain aware of the ways in which such relationships are often uneven while conducting the work. There are points where there is an attentiveness to 'building' the friendship with participants in ways that may feel natural, but remain under examined: for example, when relationships are struck through social media, which can open the door to new levels of intimacy, and vulnerability for either/both researchers.

In this case, the lead researcher, a doctoral student, is acutely aware of the distance that remains between herself and the young people, appropriately raising questions about the limits of data collection when relationships become more complex. Seeking to redress the imbalance that exists, the doctoral researcher strives to understand what the limits are of friendship and data collection opportunities. In this situation, there is room for some aspects of data collection to emerge through ethnographic strategies (participant-observation) rather than through participatory techniques such as peer research activities, including focus groups and interviews. Erring on the side of caution, this researcher creates an opportunity for community researchers to review their data and effectively choose to have their data included or removed from the analysis. This reflects the kind of on-going attempt that researchers need to make in participatory research to think through emergent ethical issues about confidentiality and privacy. Interestingly, these are different concepts which may not necessarily be fully understood, a point that is discussed in detail in Chapter 5 of this book.

Case 3.3 The power and dilemmas of 'in between' and off-the-record: Participatory research with people with intellectual disabilities in the Netherlands

Mieke Cardol

Introduction

This case example was contributed by a university researcher. It is based on her involvement in a research project in the Netherlands with and about people with intellectual disabilities. In the Netherlands, recently the support needed to participate in the community was transferred to the local municipalities.

The case

This case is about a research project that studied community participation from an experiential knowledge point of view, given the slogan of the disability studies movement: 'Nothing about us without us' and the fact that professional views and interventions until now were not able to change barriers to participation for people with intellectual disabilities. The project was carried out in the context of a Disability Studies programme and funded by a Dutch health research funding organisation (ZonMw, The Netherlands Organisation for Health Research and Development). At the time of the study, the author of this case worked at NIVEL (Netherlands Institute for Health Services Research). The study was performed in close collaboration with the Dutch self-advocacy movement of people with intellectual disabilities (LFB).

The research project focused on how people with intellectual disabilities living in the community make themselves at home in the community and what they need to do so. Nine people with intellectual disabilities were co-researchers in the project. They were recruited by the LFB and trained by a person from the LFB together with the university researchers. The interview questions were based on an adapted questionnaire about participation and empowerment ('Ask me!'), also used by the LFB. The community researchers undertook interviews in pairs with the research respondents, who were people with intellectual disabilities. The interviews were audio-recorded to limit the need to take notes in answer to the open questions. The two university researchers (junior researcher and senior researcher, author of this case) interviewed the professional supporters of the people with intellectual disabilities and the local policy officers about their strategies towards the participation of people with disabilities in the community. The university researchers also organised gatherings with the community researchers in which experiences could be shared, and dilemmas and preliminary results of the study were discussed.

The interviews with the people with intellectual disabilities took place at the respondents' homes. To get there, the community researchers had to travel by train or bus, quite far sometimes, compared with what they were used to. In all cases, the junior university researcher made the appointments for the interviews, a plan for the trip, with time tables, walking routes and street plans. Both university researchers were available to be contacted by telephone, in case something happened or was needed. Nevertheless, most community researchers wanted to travel together with one of the university researchers, as they were not used to travelling by train or bus by themselves. So, the junior researcher travelled with them, but she did not interfere in the interviews. During the interviews, she waited outside.

While travelling, the community researchers and the junior researcher talked about their lives – how they live, what friends they have or would like to have, things that make them happy or sad, experiences with attitudes of neighbours or others, etc. In fact, with regard to the research questions, the conversations during the travel brought up far more valuable information than the interviews with the respondents. Precisely the talking 'in between', the sharing of experiences, in an unforced and natural way, unintentionally worked very well.

Also at the gatherings in which the researchers practised interview techniques together, shared dilemmas regarding interviewing and discussed the preliminary results of the project, more or less the same thing happened. The community researchers added personal and important information to the interview results. From them I really learned what it meant not to feel at home in a neighbourhood, to be ignored or to be bullied. They also told us what they do to feel at home in the community. I was affected by the creativity of their strategies. For example, one community researcher reacted to the comment of an interviewee that he likes to go to the bus station, because more people are waiting there, and this provides chances to start a conversation. The community researcher agreed and added that it works to go to the bus station every week at the same time of the day to meet the same people again. These gatherings were eye-opening experiences, and moving too, because I felt I had never been so close to the lived experiences of people with intellectual disabilities.

At the end of the project, one of the community researchers asked the junior researcher to become her friend. The junior researcher was confused, as she liked the woman who asked her the question, but had not thought of her in terms of friendship. She felt the friendship could not be equal and told the community researcher that she was sorry, but she did not feel able to grant her request. The woman was very disappointed.

These experiences raised several questions for me. To begin with, how should we deal with personal data and valuable information about living with a disability gathered 'in between' and 'off the record'? We decided not to use the personal information revealed during the travelling time. But we did not want to leave it like that. Instead, we organised another focus group with the community researchers, informed them about the goal and background of the gathering, which would involve discussing the results and experiences of the respondents and evaluating whether the community researchers recognised the results as relating to their own lives. I am still not sure we did the right thing. In retrospect, I think we should have come up with a totally different study design right from the start. The focus group gathering turned the community researchers into respondents, and this was not sufficiently clear to them. At the start of the study, they were proud to be co-researchers with salaries, and they still perceived themselves and acted as such in the focus group. We, the university researchers had changed their roles, without overseeing all the consequences.

There was also another consequence: by using the personal experiences of the community researchers as data, the university researchers and two of the community researchers found they could not mention the names of the community researchers in a publication, as we feared the results could be traced to individual people. This way, we could not give credit, officially, to their work. Further, there is a dilemma concerning good participatory research. Working together and building a personal relationship is important in research like this. We, the university researchers, felt we were co-creating in a project on a basis of equality. But at the time one of the community researchers referred to this equality in the project by proposing friendship, the researcher was confronted with her thoughts about the co-researcher as someone with a disability. Should we have explicitly paid attention to the difference between a working relationship and friendship? Did we implicitly make false promises by working closely together? Or is this possibly something that can happen in every research project? Furthermore, data analyses of the last focus group discussion turned the community researchers into respondents. The transition from being community researcher to being the researched suddenly was there again. How should we deal with these multiple identities in one person? Possible differences between people should not be eliminated, but how much difference can there be, while still co-creating?

Commentary on Case 3.3

Anne MacFarlane and Brenda Roche

Case 3.3 continues the theme of blurred identities and resonates strongly with Case 3.2. In research projects, particularly participatory ones, there is an intensity and closeness that can accompany the project. As participatory research is so heavily shaped by the relationships of the partners, it is not unusual for partners to share elements of their personal lives. This can surface connections and a knowledge of one another that is beyond the scope of the research itself. As a result, this can begin to shape friendships or collegial relationships that are independent of the working roles of the project team. For all involved, these adaptations can give rise to uncertainty as the personal and the professional collide. Furthermore, co-production of knowledge is not bounded by a formal data generation encounter as in more conventional research. There are standard practices for 'opening' and 'closing' these encounters. There are guidelines for good practice in conventional qualitative research that can be referred to when 'rich data' is revealed after the tape recording has been turned off in an interview (King and Horrocks, 2010).

As in Case 3.2, the researcher in this case shows keen, critical awareness of the unintended consequences in terms of propositions of friendship. With regards to managing 'off the record' data, the researcher drew on her methodological expertise in qualitative research to design focus groups to formally record data. This too had unintended consequences in terms of further layering of community members' identities. This critical reflection from the researcher elucidates that there can be 'ripple effects of ripple effects'.

What other actions might have been taken? To maintain the integrity of the community researchers as community researchers in this kind of situation, the academic could simply choose not to use the data collected incidentally while travelling. Alternatively, they could discuss the issue that had arisen with the community researchers and offer the opportunity to come together as a co-inquiry group. This would provide a space for both academics and community researchers to more formally consider the issues that have been raised 'off the record'. Overall, this case is important because it reminds us that PR researchers need to have this commitment to reflect on participatory spaces in all their (formal and informal) shapes and guises as the relational dynamics of participatory research unfold.

Case 3.4 When research becomes a therapeutic intervention: Using PhotoVoice in an Irish hospital

Geralyn Hynes

Introduction

This case is written by an academic working in Ireland, who, with a small project group, led a PhotoVoice project involving 11 participants attending a hospital for treatment of respiratory conditions. PhotoVoice is a process that allows people to identify, represent and address issues of importance to them through photography. Typically, participants are given cameras and develop photography skills and techniques over a series of structured workshops. In the case below, PhotoVoice presented an opportunity for a participant to make meaning of her life. This raised questions about moving from PhotoVoice as a part of a research project to PhotoVoice as a therapeutic intervention, thus blurring the boundaries between research and therapy.

The case

We were a project group comprising three nurses, an artist and a nursing academic (formerly a nurse, the author of this case), who came together because of a shared interest in PhotoVoice as a means of opening conversations among health care professionals and patients about illness experiences. We gained funding from an agency connected with the hospital in which the project took place. We recruited people who were attending the hospital with different respiratory conditions, referred to here as 'participants'. We followed the structures and process for PhotoVoice projects as set out by the London-based international organisation called PhotoVoice (see www.photovoice.org).

Our aims were two-fold. First, through exhibiting the photographs generated from the project, we wanted to create a space for health care professionals coming from different disciplines (e.g. medicine, nursing, social work) to dialogue with one another. Second, we wanted to create a space for people who had a health condition to tell their stories in ways that could generate different kinds of conversations from those arising from the more usual patient experience research studies driven by the researcher's particular disciplinary lens.

The project went through the normal processes for approval from the participating hospital. Leaflets were distributed to patients attending a respiratory clinic in the hospital over a one-month period. The leaflets provided information about the project and contact details of one member of the project group. Twelve people made contact, one of whom dropped out after the first meeting because of work commitments. The remaining 11 participated in the project. All had respiratory illnesses including tuberculosis and different degrees of chronic respiratory disease. None of the participants had previously heard of PhotoVoice, nor had they experienced a participatory or action research project.

From the outset, our participants expressed their enjoyment of the project. Some teased us about our efforts to evaluate each session through structured questions. They argued that their enjoyment was self-evident and the questions were not necessary. They engaged fully in any homework that was set between group sessions. This homework initially involved taking images of shapes and angles, but then progressed on to stories. We encouraged participants to tell whatever stories they wished about themselves, rather than feeling that they should focus on their health conditions. Once they had taken their images for their stories, we then worked one-on-one with participants. This involved a project group member working with a participant to capture the essence of his/her particular story; identify the image that best reflected the story; and finally develop a caption for the image that told the story's essence.

One of the participants with whom I worked spoke about how her condition impacted on her life and family relations. We spoke at length about her illness story and her love for her family. The quality of our conversation shifted as I reflected on her emphasis on love for her family and her struggle with considerable disability arising from her condition. I was conscious that I was using skills learned from training in logotherapy (a type of psychotherapy focussing on meaning-making). However, I was also conscious that her stories and images were not finished affairs but rather her attempt to make sense of her current life, including a sense of purpose in her relations with others. I challenged her to reconcile her expressions of love with her sense of her life at this time as having little purpose. I asked her to consider how her expressions of love might be contributing to the well-being of a family member. In the end, the captions that she chose for her photographs centred on her love for her family and her struggle to survive.

The final images that this woman identified and the captions that we eventually developed reflected resilience, purpose in life and love. However, these emerged from a combination of her desire to make sense of her life and my drawing on my therapy skills to help her to achieve this desire. She did not necessarily set out to make sense of her life at the start of the project. In other words, making sense of her life was her PhotoVoice story, but one that was at least influenced by my challenging her assumptions about her life as one without purpose.

The participants subsequently exhibited their work in community and hospital settings to much acclaim. This participant brought her entire family to the exhibition launch. I was conscious that though she expressed delight in having taken part in the project, she had not signed up for conversations that exposed her deepest feelings. Whilst she had come to see her engagement with PhotoVoice as an opportunity to explore what was most meaningful for her, it is likely that my bringing my logotherapy training to bear on our conversations moved her exploration to a deep level.

In keeping with the ethical requirements for the conduct of research, a distinction is drawn between the researcher and therapist, whereby the researcher does not engage in a therapeutic relationship with the participant while wearing his/her researcher hat. If PhotoVoice is a participatory method that enables participants to make sense of their stories, then that arguably reflects a therapeutic intervention. To suggest to an ethical review board that a proposed PhotoVoice project is at once both a therapeutic intervention and research would inevitably result in rejection. The researcher is thus faced with rendering the therapeutic element a covert one in the PhotoVoice process.

Commentary on Case 3.4

Anne MacFarlane and Brenda Roche

Inclusive strategies in research connect people in ways that are often unexpected. They bridge roles and tasks in research with activities that are less conventional methods of collecting and working with data, including art-informed methods. PhotoVoice is one such approach that works to elicit perspectives and reflections through the use of photography (Wang & Burris 1997; Hergenrather et al. 2009). It is well-established as a technique in participatory research (Wang 2003), that also can have value therapeutically. The dual purpose of such a technique can be useful in drawing out key perspectives and beliefs, and as a matter of process, enabling people to reflect on and sort through tensions or unresolved issues. In this way, this case shifts our attention from ethical challenges for community researchers and academics doing participatory research, to the challenges experienced by practitioners or practitioner-academics. In this case, the author is an academic, who is also a qualified nurse and logotherapist. A key ethical dilemma is whether it is more ethical to separate or 'manage' the research and therapeutic dimensions or to celebrate the synergy and seek ways to harness both?

In Case 3.4 we see how this dilemma unfolded. For the researcher, the skillset used in research and in therapeutic work both emerge in the process of conducting a participatory Photovoice initiative. The synergies that existed between a participatory research framework and therapeutic strategies meant that the project yielded more insights than anticipated. Does this pose an ethical challenge? For the researcher, it may, as she experiences some blending of identities, tasks and activities that traditionally belong to one category versus another. For the community participant, the murkiness of roles may lead them to reveal sensitive information that they might not normally choose to as part of a research project. As a result, information that may be appropriate in a therapeutic setting can enter a domain where it unintentionally becomes research data.

The details as articulated by the researcher in Case 3.4 suggest that, in this situation, for the community participant there were no negative effects due to this merging of research and therapy. Instead, the participant felt there were additional benefits that were unanticipated but welcomed. These constitute important, although unanticipated, 'impacts', or 'ripple effects', which may be less common in traditional research, and speak to the action orientation of PR. All the same, it is worth noting that while, in this instance, participants experienced positive effects from this blurring of research and the therapeutic, there is potential for such a connection to go awry. In this case, the academic researcher was also a qualified nurse and logotherapist. This meant that participants who did reflect on sensitive aspects of their lives with her could be assumed to be relatively safe. But the case does raise an interesting question about whether, when in the role of researcher, the author of the case should also have engaged in therapy? Was she overstepping a boundary, or was she acknowledging, and utilising to good effect, her role as 'practitioner researcher'?

This potential for adverse reactions to the blending of research and therapeutic insights raises important questions for researchers that should be considered at the outset of projects. Where there may be potential for sensitive issues to emerge, should researchers have on hand connections to therapeutic supports as necessary? Does this raise, for ethical review boards, areas where they might recommend best practices for researchers to consider as 'back up' on projects?

The researcher ends the case example by asking a stark and pertinent question: should the therapeutic element of art-based methods (and potentially other methods in PR) be revealed to ethics review panels? Arguably, there is work to be done to build knowledge and understanding among ethics review panel members about the synergies that PR offers and to develop more sophisticated and nuanced guidance for the submission and review of proposals from the PR tradition.

PART 3: CONCLUDING COMMENTS

Anne MacFarlane and Brenda Roche

This chapter has focused on the ethical implications of the permeable boundaries of the roles and identities of those involved in PR. We have unpacked the notion that *boundaries are blurred* for members of participatory research teams in differing ways.

This is not problematic or challenging in and of itself. When permeable boundaries intersect with relational dynamics, however, ethical dilemmas can arise. The cases in this chapter demonstrate that this kind of intersection does happen. It is often a function of the participatory space as a fluid and open space without formal 'openings' and 'closings'. It is a space in which research partnerships are shaped by and are shaping the nature and integrity of the relationships between academic and community members as well as between community members.

This is because relationality, which is so central to PR, is about dynamics of trust, confidence and personal connection unfolding in real space and time. Finally, it is about how these dynamics are also relevant beyond the official life time of an individual project. It is important to note that the chapter has concentrated on cases about community and academic relationships. Much PR can be based on partnerships between community and academic partners working alongside health services or planners, which is likely to have some shared and differential issues that are worth investigating. In health and social care, such research is emerging more and more. This increasingly involves networks of service users and advocates, as well as policy-makers and decision-makers, within a system where interests may be shared about generating certain forms of evidence, or in moving towards key action points. However, the nature of what these partnerships look like from the perspective of roles and relationships remains less examined, and often, poorly articulated. This can surface a host of ethical challenges, some of which have been considered in this chapter. What the boundaries of researcher and co-researchers' roles look like when we focus on more socio-political interests may be very different from some of the lines blurred around social relationships. As public and private partnerships are increasingly explored, and drawing on the use of participatory methods, the nature of such relationships and how roles and interests may blur warrants further examination, and ethical consideration.

The implications of the analysis presented in this chapter are that we need to acknowledge the relational nature of participatory research as a strength and an area of potential tension. There is an opportunity and responsibility to add to the existing literature to make this overt through critical reflection and empirical analyses. These, in turn, can be used to add depth, nuance and strength to training initiatives for PR and the practice of ethical review boards. It is also essential, however, to create spaces that support PR projects to explore how the core values of PR are enacted in real space and time and to consider, from the stance of covenantal ethics, what response is appropriate in real space and time.

References

Banks, S., Armstrong, A., Carter, K., Graham, H., Hayward, P., Henry, A., . . . & Moore, N. (2013). Everyday ethics in community-based participatory research. *Contemporary Social Science*, 8(3), 263–277.

Brydon-Miller, M. (2009). Covenantal ethics and action research: Exploring a common foundation for social research. In D. Mertens & P. Ginsberg (Eds.), *Handbook of social research ethics* (pp. 243–258). Newbury Park, CA: SAGE.

Canadian Institute of Health Research (2007). *Guidelines for Health Research with Aboriginal Communities*. Ottawa, Canada: CIHR.

Chambers R. (2002). *Participatory Workshops: a Sourcebook of 21 Sets of Ideas and Activities*. New York: Routledge.

Flicker, S., Roche, B., & Guta, A. (2010). *Peer research in action III: Ethical issues*. Toronto: Wellesley Institute.

Goodson L. and Phillimore J. (eds) (2012). *Community research for participation: From theory to method*. Bristol: Policy Press.

Greene, S. (2013). Peer research assistantships and the ethics of reciprocity in community-based research. *Journal of Empirical Research on Human Research Ethics*, 8(2), 141–152.

Greene, S., Ahluwalia, A., Watson, J., Tucker, R., Rourke, S. B., Koornstra, J., . . . & Byers,

S. (2009). Between skepticism and empowerment: the experiences of peer research assistants in HIV/AIDS, housing and homelessness community-based research. *International Journal of Social Research Methodology, 12*(4), 361–373.

Greenhalgh T., Voisey C. and Robb, N. (2007) Interpreted consultations as 'Business as usual': An analysis of Organisational Routines. *Sociology of Health and Illness 29*(6), 931–954.

Hart, A. and Aumann, K. (2012) Challenging inequalities through community-university partnerships. In Benneworth, P (Ed.) *University Engagement with Socially Excluded Communities* (pp. 47–65). Dordrecht: Springer.

Hergenrather, K.C., Rhodes, S.D., Cowan, C.A., Pula, S (2009). Photovoice as Community-Based Participatory Research: A Qualitative Review. *American Journal of Health Behaviour 33*(6), 686–698.

International Collaboration for Participatory Health Research (ICPHR) (2013). *Position Paper (1), What is Participatory Health Research?* Berlin: ICPHR, www.icphr.org/uploads/2/0/3/9/20399575/ichpr_position_paper_1_defintion_-_version_may_2013.pdf (accessed 31 October 2017).

King, N. and Horrocks, C. (2010). *Interviews in Qualitative Research.* Los Angeles: SAGE.

Kothari ,U. (2001) Power, knowledge and social control in participatory development. In: B. Cooke and U. Kothari (Eds.) *Participation: the New Tyranny?* (pp. 139–152). London: ZED Books.

MacFarlane, A., Dzebisova. Z., Karapish. D., Kovacevic, B. Ogbebor, F., & Okonkwo, E. (2009) Arranging and negotiating the use of informal interpreters in general practice consultations: experiences of refugees and asylum seekers in the west of Ireland. *Social Science and Medicine 69*(2), 210–214.

McLaughlin, H. (2005). Young service users as co-researchers: Methodological problems and possibilities. *Qualitative Social Work, 4*(2), 211–228.

Mosavel, M., Ahmed, R., Daniels, D., & Simon, C. (2011). Community researchers conducting health disparities research: Ethical and other insights from fieldwork journaling. *Social Science & Medicine, 73*(1), 145–152.

Mosavel, M., & Sanders, K. D. (2014). Community-engaged research: cancer survivors as community researchers. *Journal of Empirical Research on Human Research Ethics, 9*(3), 74–78.

O'Reilly-de Brún, M, de Brún, T., O'Donnell, C.A. et al. (2017). Material practices for meaningful engagement: An analysis of participatory learning and action research techniques for data generation and analysis in a health research partnership. *Health Expectations,* https://doi.org/10.1111/hex.12598

O'Reilly-de Brún, M., de Brún, T., Okonkwo, E., Bonsenge-Bokanga, J.-S., De Almeida Silva, M.M., Ogbebor, F., Mierzejewska, A., Nnadi, L., van Weel-Baumgarten, E., van Weel, C., van den Muijsenbergh, M. and MacFarlane, A. (2016) 'Using Participatory Learning & Action research to access and engage with 'hard to reach' migrants in primary healthcare research', *BMC Health Services Research, 16*(1), 25.

Richman, K. A., Alexander, L. B., & True, G. (2012). Proximity, ethical dilemmas, and community research workers. *AJOB Primary Research, 3*(4), 19–29.

Richman, K. A., Alexander, L. B., & True, G. (2015). How Do Street-Level Research Workers Think About the Ethics of Doing Research "On the Ground" With Marginalized Target Populations? *AJOB Empirical Bioethics, 6*(2), 1–11.

Roche, B. (2008). *New directions in community-based research.* Toronto, ON: Wellesley Institute.

Roche, B., Flicker, S., & Guta, A. (2010). *Peer research in action I: models of practice.* Toronto, ON: Wellesley Institute.

True, G., Alexander, L. B., & Fisher, C. B. (2017). Supporting the role of community members employed as research staff: Perspectives of community researchers working in addiction research. *Social Science & Medicine, 187,* 67–75.

van den Muijsenbergh, M., van Weel-Baumgarten, E., Burns, N., O'Donnell. C., Mair, F., Spiegel, W., et al. (2014). Communication in cross-cultural consultations in primary care in Europe: the case for improvement. The rationale for the RESTORE FP 7 project. *Primary Health Care Res Dev., 15*(2), 122–133.

Wang, C. (2003). Using photo voice as a participatory assessment and issue selection tool. In M. Minkler and N. Wallerstein (Eds,) *Community-based participatory research for health* (pp. 179–196). San Francisco, CA: John Wiley & Sons.

Wang, C, & Burris, M.A. (1997). Photovoice: concept, methodology, and use for participatory needs assessment. *Health Education & Behavior, 24*(3), 369–387.

Warr, D., Mann, R., & Williams, R. (2012). Avoiding 'best' being the enemy of 'good': Using peer interviewer methods for community research in place-based settings in Australia. In Goodson, L., & Phillimore, J. (Eds.), *Community research for participation: From theory to method* (pp. 215–231). Chicago, IL: The Policy Press.

4

COMMUNITY RIGHTS, CONFLICT AND DEMOCRATIC REPRESENTATION

Meghna Guhathakurta

With cases contributed by Monika Bjeloncikova, Shaun Cleaver, Angela Contreras, Vendula Gojova and Michael J. Kral

PART 1: INTRODUCTION AND OVERVIEW OF ISSUES

Meghna Guhathakurta

This chapter raises some core ethical issues that lie at the heart of community-based participatory research (PR). It foregrounds the tensions between the collective and the individual, the 'insider' and 'outsider' viewpoints, inter-community and intra-community conflict and issues of representation in democratic contexts. The cases that elucidate these dynamics in Part 2 of the chapter traverse a wide range of global regions, cultural contexts and diversities and yet dwell on ethical concerns that have commonalities and are shared the world over. It is through this lens of shared experience that I have tried to address some of the core ethical concerns that the authors of the cases have highlighted. Although I do not belong to any of the regions or cultural contexts depicted by the four cases, my experiences of participatory action research with marginalised communities through Research Initiatives, Bangladesh (RIB), my own experiences in feminist research practices as well as university education are implicated in the comments I have to offer.

The chapter first delineates the areas mentioned in the title: community rights, conflict and democratic representation with a view to engage issues and perspectives related to ethical aspects of participatory research. From this engagement the discussions evolve around certain principles that are relevant to the cases. In Case 4.1 from Canada an adult education practitioner and scholar reflects on her experiential learning and tensions that stemmed out of being an advocate for low-waged Temporary Foreign Workers (TFWs), a student researcher, and volunteer at a church group. Case 4.2 was contributed by a Canadian working with a community of persons with disability in rural Zambia, which raised questions about how to deal with issues of power and privilege between leaders and other members of the community. Case 4.3 relates to the study of suicide and well-being among the Inuit in Nunavut Arctic Canada. The researcher considered it to be a case of power and privilege concerning gender, age and ethnicity raising questions about individual versus collective behaviour, personality and positionality. Case 4.4 was contributed by two university researchers involved in community-based participatory research in an officially designated 'socially excluded locality' in the Czech Republic. This case highlights the ethnic tensions in such localities and the potential for conflict, confusion, and disputes when university researchers attempt to engage with exist-ing community workers and community groups. The case illustrates ethical issues of institutional involvement, inter-sectionality and intra-group conflicts that often accompany PR.

In all four cases some ethical concerns were raised by the researchers themselves, but others were inherent in the research design and pedagogic approaches that were adopted. Questions of ethics were raised around issues of silence, gender and racial prejudices, social stigma and positionality of the researchers with respect to their beliefs and commitment. Confronted with these challenges the researchers sought to resolve them in innovative ways, often alone, at other times informed through their partners in research or supervisors. Whatever the research outcome, the cases reveal important lessons to be learnt in the field of PR on questions of ethics.

I will now discuss some of the concepts and themes that may help to make sense of the cases in Part 2.

Community rights

The concept of community rights stems from the strands of community develop-ment practices that have evolved over the years. As a response to the critique of top-down approaches model, community development emphasised the perspec-tive of the local community in the development process. The varied models that evolved from these trends have been characterised in different ways:

(a) *Large-scale versus small-scale.* This contrasts those projects needing high levels of technology as inputs and sustenance, such as practices by international institu-tions such as World Bank and IMF, and those emphasising simple technologies managed by local people.
(b) *Specialised versus comprehensive.* Specialised forms necessitate experts and focus on one group or one sector while comprehensive forms would combine and coordinate more holistic processes of development.
(c) *Needs-based versus asset-based.* This distinguishes processes where the local people are mere passive recipients of the development and do not partake in its solution, whereas asset-based processes underline the mobilisation of such inherent assets that the community may possess (see Stoecker, 2014).

Community rights have featured in the empowerment-oriented models more so than the technocratic ones. The UK House of Commons Communities and

Local Government Committee report on Community Rights (2015) brings out strongly the asset-based approach to community development where it reviews the UK government's policy of empowering people through the establishment of community rights to save local assets from closure, build community housing, take over local authority services and bring public land back into use (Communities and Local Government Committee, 2015).

These varied notions of community development and rights foreground two discourses that relate directly to participatory research and the ethics of such research. One is embedded in the notion of participation, the other in notions of individual versus community rights.

As the grassroots model of community gained predominance, the question of participation became more intense. How was such participation from the local community to take place in the structures that were set up? Who actually participated and what was the nature of such participation? The Institute of Development Studies at the University of Sussex led this discussion and books such as *Participation, the New Tyranny* (Cooke & Kothari, 2001) questioned some of the lip service and tokenism inherent in such participatory practices. Non-governmental organisations (NGOs) that genuinely worked with people at the grassroots and advocated participatory practices adopted the stance that participatory development in order to be meaningful needed to be "for the people, of the people and indeed by the people" (internal communication with Misereor, a German church-based aid agency). Whilst the first two were often inscribed into the agenda of many NGOs and community-based organisations (CBOs), it was the third tenet ('by the people') that proved to be the most challenging. Raising the ethical questions in participatory research also treads similar paths. In many cases research was conducted taking into consideration the involvement and perspectives of people or people's representatives, but fell short of involving them in the actual design of the research or project, which was left to experts and/or academics.

This brings us to the second area of discourse that problematises the notion of community itself. Two questions arise in participatory research: (a) How does one balance individual rights with community rights (Goldfarb & Shamoo, 2008); and (b) How does one address inter-community and intra-community conflict and relations? Such discourses also lead us to the area of our second notion, i.e. conflict.

Much has been written on the issue of individual versus community/collective rights, especially in the field of human rights and the debate about cultural relativism. Whereas classically human rights are constructed as universal individual rights, cultural relativism asserts that human values emerge in social, cultural, religious, economic and political contexts and therefore differ from one community to the next (Donnelly, 1984; Vasilache, 2009). This has brought in a lively debate between human rights as perceived in the developed North and developing South and the right to cultural freedom has been articulated and pitched against universal standards and norms foregrounding many debates regarding segregation of women and gender equality. In such debates it is again the notion of participation and voice that has been engaged. Whose voices articulate cultural freedom? Are they the elites of the community or the subalterns? Are they men or women? Ideally participatory action research is designed to engage multiple voices within a community and address any intra-community conflict therein. The recording of differences and exceptions are just as important as consensus and norms that guide the collective or 'common good'.

Conflict

The variegated nature of the community naturally leads us to an area where PR encounters conflict: between the individual and community, between members of the same community, and between one community and another or community and the state.

Conflict is often seen as integral to society. Many theorists such as Karl Marx consider conflict, particularly class conflict, to be necessary for the evolution of society. Others such as Lester Ward and Ludwig Gumplowicz (Ward, 1909; Ward & Gumplowicz, 1971) take a comprehensive anthropological and evolutionary point of view and posit that civilisation has been shaped by conflict between cultures and ethnic groups.

In the above section too we see that PR encounters conflicts both within and outside communities. However the issue here is related to the role that PR should play in encountering and engaging in such conflicts. Engaging with conflict foregrounds three different approaches either from action researchers or actors in the field. These are (a) conflict management, (b) conflict resolution, and (c) conflict transformation. Each of these notions is embedded in a rich literature, but generally one can characterise them as follows: conflict management is functional and managerial in focus. Managing conflict that emerges out of competitive interests may entail mediation by a third party. Conflict resolution deals with problems that arise out of unfulfilled or frustrated human needs between two or more parties and hence aims to reach solutions of such needs. Conflict transformation takes place when confrontations between people are seen as a result of disempowerment and injustice and hence addressing such conflicts assumes the transformation of such structures. This entails a more deep-rooted and long-term process for which PR is particularly amenable (Rothman, 2014).

Participatory research may address all three processes depending on the nature of the conflict and the time available to each researcher/animator to address these conflicts, but the third one regarding conflict transformation necessitates longerterm processes and skillful facilitation. Here the process needs to be owned by the parties in question and entails engagement with both community voices as well as society at large.

Democratic representation

Nation-states *per se* need not be democratic, as the world realised with the rise of the fascist state, but a key distinction of a democratic nation-state is the identification of a *people* with a *polity* within it. One of the relationships this polity can have with the power that controls the state is embedded in the very notion of democracy – literally being ruled by the people.

But the practice of democracy does not always take place on a level playing field, benefitting all segments of the population equally; vast inequalities of power and resources may separate the haves and have-nots. Therefore systems and practices of democracy also vary. The pluralist version of democracy – where power is a result of open competition, there are fair winners and losers, and the public arena is free and equal – exists mostly in theory. The second form of democracy is the elitist version, or what Marxists call the bourgeois democracy, where power is maintained through systemic discrimination and privilege, where people need clout, bargaining skills, and resources to win, and power is conflictual. Then, there is the ideological version, or majoritarianism, where power is maintained through ideological (mostly of the majority) values, institutional barriers to inclusiveness remain in both the public and private arena, and hegemony – which incorporates both consensus and repression – prevents conflicts from arising (Gaventa, 1995).

It is within these different concepts of democracy that one can also delineate the spaces of inequality and violence. In the first category, free societies are not necessarily equal or fair ones. Free competition means the survival of the fittest, and hence the society becomes divided into achievers and losers. The spaces of violence in such societies therefore lie in the absence of protective measures for the weak. The term 'bourgeois democracy', used to describe the second category, emerges as a critique of the first. Inequality among classes is considered to be part of the structure, and hence the violence that takes place between the haves and have-nots is also structural and thus is inherent in such systems. In this category violence results when policies favour the majority and exclude the minority. The latter two systems indicate and implicate spaces of violence which may affect citizenship for all as a result of exclusionary politics of the state. Taken to the extreme, this may lead to forced migration or flight from the home country (Rohmann, 1999).

The relationship between democracy and citizenship is therefore crucial to consider. Citizenship is the status of a person recognised by custom or law as being a member of a state. A person may have multiple citizenships, and a person who does not have citizenship of any state is said to be stateless. But this is merely the outward aspect of citizenship. Citizenship can be passive, as in merely obeying the laws of the state in exchange for enjoying protection from it, or it can mean an active participation in public life and democratic processes. This is often distinguished as the liberal, individual conception of democracy in the first instance and the civic, participatory democracy in the second. In modern-day democracies, the first idea of citizenship is more common at the national level where the social contract theory is directly applicable, whilst at the local level – i.e., town councils, city corporations, or rural governing bodies – the second notion has more propensity to prevail. It is also at the local level that it can be detected whether citizenship truly manifests itself or not by overriding and going beyond bonds of kinship (reminiscent of feudal ties) to unite people with different backgrounds (class, gender, religion, caste, race) into one inclusive body politic (Gaventa, 1995).

Citizenship may involve the proactive response of citizens in the formulation of the system's structures and its rules. Denial of such space to people whose voices are not yet articulated but are likely to be heard in the future may form the roots of violence, which may manifest itself in exclusionary policies, racial profiling or discriminatory laws. The politics of voice that is embedded in PR is therefore crucial in understanding true democratic representation.

The issue of voice and representation is raised in elucidating the general principles of community dialogue that are relevant to our discussion. The principles are (a) deep democracy and (b) deep multiculturalism.

Deep democracy indicates processes and mechanisms which enable the voices of a wide range of people in a community to be heard, not just those who form the majority, or the mainstream. Deep democracy is therefore characterised by the legitimisation of diverse interests, full transparency, listening and well-informed decision-making according to criteria that are explicit and clear to all (Shemer, 2014).

Deep multiculturalism implies the creation of a public space where different communities or groups interact with each other from the perspective of their own cultural identity. This is therefore not a neutral given space, but one that needs to be co-constructed through open discussion, negotiation and decision-making according to criteria that are explicit and clear to all actors (Shemer, 2014). This is where PR comes into play.

Ethical issues in PR

I have briefly sketched the different notions under discussion in this chapter and related them to PR. I now take some points from this discussion to illustrate how these factors relate to issues of ethics in PR. These talking points can be categorised in the following way:

(a) The ethics of silence and voice
(b) Positionality and its impact on the researcher
(c) Intersectionality and intra-group conflicts
(d) The prerogative of the institution

(a) The ethics of silence and voice

Patricia Lundy and Mark McGovern (2006), in 'The ethics of silence: Action research, community 'truth-telling' and post-conflict transition in the North of Ireland' state, "The position that researchers take when faced with an ethical dilemma is likely to be affected by their motivation for doing the research, its purpose, and whom they see benefitting from it" (p. 51). Because PR is a method that is considered especially sensitive to community-based truth-telling, the ethics of preserving silence or giving voice is a dilemma that faces most researchers, particularly those who work in conflict or post-conflict zones. The aim of the researcher is ultimately to engage in a process informed by a participatory action research approach and hence a community-based form of truth-telling can act as the means to permit previously unheard voices to emerge into the public realm and so help shape the future in a public way (Lundy & McGovern, 2006).

However, going into a discursive practice in a conflict-ridden zone is far from being a smooth journey and this relates to any kind of conflict even in times of peace. The researcher has to weigh carefully the *costs* of truth-telling against its ultimate benefits for individuals and society at large. Often it is has to do with the protection of the individual or collective from immediate harm. For example, in Bangladesh, Research Initiatives, Bangladesh (RIB) supported a local group that practised interactive theatre on the theme of rape of a village girl and got to know that both the parents of the girl and some of the rapists (who were sons of powerful villagers and hence had escaped being caught) were actually in the audience. The animator had to stop the parents from speaking out the truth in public, as they would then be endangered. The facilitator instead allowed the airing of emotions to take place in an impersonal way. Following this, in order to serve the cause of justice, the theatre group did report the incident to the local government officials and requested them to take up the matter with the police. That was just about all they could do in the circumstances.

Whether it is peace-building, conflict transformation or confidence building, time and process are of the utmost importance. One cannot rush into these things and it must be remembered that PR is only one of the entry points for such processes to begin. The ethics of such a process must include a constant process of praxis (Rahman, 1994), i.e., action reflection, action by the participants and this is what the researcher should leave behind in the community, well beyond the period of the actual research itself. Lundy and McGovern conclude from an evaluation of their research project that 'the best means of dealing with the ethical problems of sensitivity and danger was to ensure that those taking part understood precisely what the project was for, felt a sense of ownership and agency over its outcomes, and could directly shape and control their deeply personal and often emotionally difficult involvement in it' (2006, p. 62).

(b) Positionality and its impact on the researcher

The issues of community, conflict and democratic representation bear heavily down on the action researcher as the research process in PR traverses terrains of inter-subjectivities, i.e., interaction which is not merely a two-way phenomenon but engages first, second and third party narratives in criticality of thinking or reviewing received notions of thought (Louis, 2014). Most PR researchers enter the research process with a predetermined positionality of engagement that can include feminism, socialism or even just the will to do good for society. Such subjective stances need not be negative for the research outcomes so long as researchers are deeply involved in self-conscious pedagogic learning throughout the research process. Nimat Hafez Barazangi writes: 'to attain equilibrium between my individual autonomy and collective social justice . . . without integrating my scholarship-activism as a Muslim woman with being a reflective AR practitioner, I would not have been able to experience the integrative ethical pedagogy that I am theorising here' (2006, p. 106).

A self-reflective sense of individual autonomy should therefore be nurtured as part of pedagogic practice. In order to achieve such equilibrium between individual autonomy and collective social justice it is necessary to inform and sensitise both impersonal and hierarchical academic settings as well as critique and interrogate pedagogies such as feminist education that both foster and undermine autonomy at the same time, often by not recognising the diverse cultural spaces that may inform one's individualities in the first instance. The challenge therefore becomes how to encourage autonomy of the individual and argue against traditional structural injustice.

(c) Intersectionality and intra-group conflicts

The question of representation emerges as an ethical issue in PR when the process or outcome of the research raises the following questions: Who is the community? Who defines the community? Does the community constitute a monolithic whole? Whose voice is heard as being representative of the community and whose is not? What does this have to say about representation and democratic practices?

In social science, communitarian principles which emphasise mutual co-operation among members of any community have both been acclaimed as well as problematised. PR is no exception to this rule. Community-based participatory research is beneficial when communitarian principles are accepted and integrated with the lifestyle of communities. But then almost all societies are in transition, and differences do arise in the conduct of daily life and the pursuit of individual welfare. One of the ways in which other trends of social science research have overcome monolithic or binary tendencies in defining the collective is to incorporate intersectionality, i.e. enabling transcendence of both individual and collective boundaries through exploring multiple dimensions of identity. Through intersectional approaches one can also take into cognisance power differentials that may reside within one community that may often lead to intra-community conflicts as is evident in Case 4.2 and Case 4.4 elaborated here. PR practitioners are, in fact, in an advantageous position to embrace intersectionality in their pedagogy as per the Tagorian principles of self-development (*atma-shakti)* combined with cooperative strength (*shakti-shamavay*) (Guhathakurta, forthcoming).

In cases of intra-group conflicts, which often influence the research outcome, it is perhaps best for the practitioner of PR to acknowledge such differences. These may be based on power differentials in society and practitioners need to acknowledge the fact that such differentials will not go away at the drop of a hat. In fact, what will be good to conclude would be to aim at the ownership of the process by all sections of the society in the long term and to engage in a way that leaves behind a legacy of practice (or praxis) in which this could be brought about.

Let me provide an example from the work of RIB in a community of pig-rearers called the Kawras living in the remote villages of Bangladesh. The Kawras are considered social outcastes and untouchable in the Hindu religious structure and in a Muslim majority society they are socially stigmatised, as pigs are considered 'haram' in the Islamic religious discourse. Therefore they could be considered to be one of the most discriminated against and marginalised communities in Bangladesh. When RIB started to work with them our animators thought it would be plain sailing. But soon the animators found that it was not easy to get any consensus from such a group. The reasons were that even though we saw them as a collective entity, they were actually divided into two distinct groups, one group owned the pigs, and the others grazed the pigs. The problems of the grazers were often caused by the owners, who did not pay them sufficiently nor took care of their health services in cases of sickness or injury. The ethical consideration for the animator was whether s/he should divide the groups into two and hence create an even deeper divide between the two groups in a community that was already isolated and stigmatised. After much discussion with fellow animators and with participants it was decided to keep them as one group but to introduce topics of discussion that concerned the whole group first, e.g. access to government services including health benefits, and to bring up more divisive issues later like wages when the groups became more sensitised to each other.

(d) The prerogative of the institution

Researchers hosted by an educational or administrative institution encounter ethical questions when it comes to choosing between their institutional prerogative and that of the participant researchers. Such institutional prerogatives of the researcher often clash with the participatory processes or lie hidden behind the tensions that are inherent in the process. Where the institution is educational, and operates outside its immediate surroundings, there is an added imperative that the good cooperative relationship between the institution and the community should not be disrupted. This often prevents a deepening of the research agenda in the event that the access gained by the researcher or future researchers would be hampered. It can also mean a loss of degree for the researcher.

The problem is even more complicated when more than one institution is involved, as the researchers may have to negotiate community or professional organisations in order to access communities. In Case 4.1, for example, the researcher had to work through a church-led organisation which worked with low-waged temporary foreign workers (TFW) who were mostly male farm hands. Here the researcher had to meet the prerogatives of a second institution, the church and its leadership when she tried to address the problem of the TFW and which in turn gave rise to several ethical issues. In order to minimise the interpretation and negotiating of values between institutions and participants by the individual researcher, ethical issues of research therefore need to be dealt with from the very outset. The ideal place where it can begin is, of course, the university or research institution itself. As Barazangi comments, 'when action researchers become educators, they too often fall short . . . they fail to develop a substantial educational framework built on AR [action research] pedagogy, AR evaluation models, and a moral compass for guiding the process' (2006, p. 98). From the perspective of the researcher she says 'without more formalised understandings and a self-conscious pedagogy, collaborators (of PR) are left to rely on their intuitiveness, leading learners to determine the authenticity of a principle vis a vis the variations of its interpretation, and social application' (p. 98).

Having outlined some of the main areas of ethical conflict within and between communities, Part 2 of the chapter presents the four cases from research practice, followed by commentaries from my perspective as a participatory researcher.

PART 2: CASES AND COMMENTARIES

Case 4.1 Doing research, advocating for human rights, and preserving community relations amongst migrant workers in Canada: A silence that (still) bothers

Angela Contreras

Introduction

This case is contributed by an adult education practitioner and scholar. It reflects on her experiential learning and tensions that stemmed out of being an advocate for low-waged temporary foreign workers (TFWs), a student researcher, and volunteer at a church group. With the approval from her university and the consent from the group's leader, the researcher studied the development of the group. TFWs employed in low-wage occupations such as nannies, janitors, and fast-food servers have precarious migration and employment status in Canada; they are vulnerable to the violation of their legal and human rights. The immigration status of these TFWs prohibits them from accessing publicly funded support and immigrant settlement services. However, organised diasporas and churches, in collaboration with community-based legal clinics, have stepped up to deliver language and culturally appropriate projects that help TFWs learn about their legal and social rights.

The case

Reverend R had just arrived in town and was looking to engage his parish in supporting migrant workers in accordance with the teachings of his religion. Upon meeting him I explained that though I didn't fully identify with his religious beliefs, I respected them and wanted to collaborate with him in developing a public legal information clinic for migrant workers. Rev. R accepted my offer and organised a space at the parish where I could work.

The group lacked a name and a formal plan, but according to Rev. R the group had a two-fold purpose: to increase the number of Spanish-speaking parishioners by providing them with meaningful volunteer opportunities at the service of vulnerable migrants, and to deliver outreach and support to migrant workers. My work at the parish corresponded to the latter purpose, but I was also happy to be part of group activities, as these could inform my study.

Unlike other pastors at the parish, Rev. R's Latin-American background helped him connect with immigrants from Spanish-speaking countries. All members of the group were originally from Latin America, and almost naturally the group oriented itself to serve Spanish-speaking migrant workers. This implied reaching out to TFWs employed as seasonal agricultural workers; they all were men and almost nearly all were from Mexico and Central America. Affectionately, the group declared that these TFWs would be "our *muchachos*" (our boys). Rev. R petitioned the group to "visit our *muchachos*, share a meal with them, let them know they are not alone." I wanted to understand how the visits helped the TFWs and how the group benefited from their volunteering. In my interviews with Rev. R and the group they asserted they knew many TFWs suffer various forms of exploitation and illegalities. A member of the group explained that visits to the farms were a good way to talk and practice compassion in a safe and respectful way because 'employers won't let their workers be visited by anyone looking for trouble, but employers are OK with our visits because we are with the church'.

At the information office progress was slow. I was struggling with recruiting and retaining volunteers, and was happy when at last a certified paralegal came to volunteer. Soon we had more TFWs wanting help than we could possibly serve at the office. Sadly, weeks later the paralegal phoned me to announce she wasn't coming back to the office. She reported to me that she grew uncomfortable working in the parish where older pastors were rude to some of her client TFWs. Matters worsened weeks later when the parish transferred Rev. R to another country, which resulted in the information clinic being shut down. Rev. L, one of the older pastors, took over the group and restructured it. The parish allowed me to continue doing my study and let me volunteer as a farm visitor.

During one of my visits to the farms I noticed that some of the *muchachos* showed skin and eye irritations which they said resulted from their exposure to chemicals at work. They explained to me they would like to seek medical treatment but were afraid their employer would not give his permission to possibly missing work time to go see a doctor. Back at the parish I suggested the group could partner with Project S. I had worked with Project S in the past; it delivers outreach and legal and health information for women TFWs. I, however, omitted to tell the group that some of the women served by Project S are sex workers.

The church group invited to one of its meetings a representative from Project S. During her presentation the guest explained that her organisation has volunteer lawyers and health professionals experienced at serving women TFWs including nannies and sex workers. She added that her association would be happy to have their professionals accompany the group in visiting the farms; in return the group would be welcome to do outreach to Spanish-speaking women TFWs.

When the guest finished her presentation Rev. L thanked her for her time and then asserted that the group exists only to support the spiritual and social needs of its members and of the men at the farms. Next, Rev. L advised the guest that if they needed Spanish-speaking volunteers then they better go to talk to women's groups at other churches.

After the guest had gone, the pastor instructed the group not to follow-up with Project S. Neither I nor anyone from the group said anything to Rev. L. We all listened to him preaching to us: 'don't let our mission be distracted by political agendas. We exist to serve the *muchachos*; they need us, they have made enormous sacrifices and are alone in this country working decent jobs so they can give their families back home a decent life.'

A few days later I resigned from the group and submitted to Rev. L my written preliminary assessment of the group's activities during my time as volunteer. I could have spoken truth to power in my report by problematising the pastor's position regarding a prospective collaboration with Project S. However, I wanted to preserve my academic relationship with the group and finish my study. I remained silent.

I regret I made the wrong call at facilitating an encounter between these two groups in hopes that it would be productive for all parties involved and for my study as well. Was my silence implying one sector of society is more deserving than another of liberation from systemic oppression?

I have not yet reached closure in regard to the silence I kept at that meeting and in my report to the church group. The silence of the members of the group and of the visitor I understand. But I am still struggling to understand why I didn't speak out and dare to tell the pastor he should open up his group to the other migrant workers' advocates.

Commentary on Case 4.1

Meghna Guhathakurta

This is a case that has haunted me quite a bit, almost as much as it seems to have haunted the researcher herself as is evident in her title. It has been written in a very frank and open manner and has graphically illustrated the complexities that one encounters in PR. The case is especially interesting as the research is located in a multilayered institutional set up ranging from the university to a church-led working group to the participants on the ground who are Temporary Foreign Workers. Problems of democratic space exist in each layer which impacts on the nature of participation that the researcher is able to generate. She also has to negotiate and interpret principles between various institutions in which she is not the prime decision-maker. On top of it all are the sensibilities that construct her own positionality: her commitment to social and feminist goals of equality. One cannot but sympathise with her and yet one could also wish that she had received the support and guidance from her colleagues and supervisors on her suggestions to involve yet another institution into play that set up a complicated dynamics of its own, i.e. the inter-institutional politics between church and the feminist organisation suggested by the researcher. The other thing that comes through her narrative is just how important it is for institutions involved in PR to keep referring to the core group of participants, in this case the TFWs, in every step of the research. The complication in this case was that their representation in the church volunteers' group was weak and hence they did not seem to have any decision-making capacity on issues that concerned them, something that the researcher tried to bridge but failed. The attempt to do so however must be commended.

Case 4.2 Whose voice is included and whose should be loudest? Negotiating value systems with respect to leadership and membership in rural Zambia

Shaun Cleaver

Introduction

I am a White, cisgender heterosexual male, non-disabled, Canadian, writing about my experience as a PhD student conducting research on disability in rural Zambia. In this qualitative research with participatory elements, I sought to better understand how Zambians with disabilities: 1) make sense of disability, and 2) frame strategies to improve the situation of persons with disabilities. As per the PhD programme requirements, I designed the study prior to the start of fieldwork, but with the intent that the participating disability groups could increasingly influence the research and its action components as the project progressed.

The case

In order to pursue my PhD dissertation research in rural Zambia, a collaborating government department introduced me to a loosely organised group of persons with disabilities. The government department officers and people in the community presented the structure of this group in inconsistent ways that were confusing to me, as an outsider. For example, the membership numbers were alternatively presented as 12, a few dozen, and over 100. In contrast to the elusive structure of the "entire group," there were nine individuals who were consistently identified as leaders. As per the study design, I worked with the leaders to prepare focus group discussions and individual interviews with group members.

In working with the leaders I began to see these nine individuals according to two profiles. The first profile applied to the four men who were considered community elders (ages 65–84). During the preparatory meetings, it was these elderly men who spoke the most among the leaders. These men repeatedly presented the challenges that they saw in the community, rather than discuss the preparation of study activities. The second profile of leader included three younger men (ages 40–55) and two women (ages 36 and 69). The leaders in the second profile were deferential to the first in multiple ways. The deferential dynamics included speaking privileges (who speaks most and when), seating arrangements (who gets chairs), and greeting obligations (who approaches; who bows or kneels). During the preparatory meetings, the leaders of the second profile spoke less, but when they did speak they spoke more about the ways that we could prepare for the study activities.

The preparatory meetings were frustrating for me. I had presented this project as simultaneous knowledge generation and social action, and participants had agreed to this at the time of recruitment. However, when planning the actual study activities it seemed that the elderly men, the 'leaders of the leaders', did not understand the importance of knowledge generation to my involvement in the community. Meanwhile, there seemed to be leaders who grasped my need to progress the research, but these leaders recognised and accepted subordinate roles in our planning discussions.

In my role as a student researcher striving for a positive impact on social justice, I pursued this work with the foundational philosophy that the project could bring voice to Zambian society's most marginalised citizens by encouraging a participatory mechanism for them to influence policy and programme changes. At the same time, I wanted to respect and support pre-existing structures. It seemed to me that these two foundational goals were in tension: the apparent pre-existing structure was one in which four senior leaders spoke on behalf of the community, possibly subjugating the voices of the most marginalised members of this already marginalised group. From this position, every potential route forward would compromise at least one foundational goal; every route forward entailed some degree of risk.

Despite the perils of moving forward, I was conducting this project as part of a PhD, and that role was not well-served by me standing still. After lengthy discussions with my supervisors about the advantages and pitfalls of various options, I unilaterally decided to redesign the data collection activities such that it was only the nine leaders who were research participants. This strategy was a practical compromise that allowed me to simplify the process of data collection and demonstrate my support for the status of the leaders. Conversely, this decision changed the role of the group leaders with respect to the project, significantly reducing their opportunities to contribute to the project's design. This decision also meant excluding from direct participation the majority of the community's members. According to my previously stated foundational goals, this compromise meant that community members had fewer opportunities for participation than foreseen while I approached the established leadership structure in a different way than it presented itself, by approaching all leaders as equals.

At the time of my departure from fieldwork, I left asking myself about the implications of my unilateral decision. Could I have amplified the difference of power and privilege between the leaders and other community members? Would there be unforeseen implications of disregarding the leadership hierarchy? Could I have negatively affected the possibility of future engagement in the community? If I did return, would I be able to negotiate new arrangements with this community that were more inclusive of all members and particularly welcoming to leadership engagement for collective benefits?

Ultimately, I successfully completed my thesis research within the allotted time of my PhD programme, and I was able to self-fund a return trip to Zambia two and a half years after the fieldwork period. Most of the faces that I saw on the return were the same ones I knew from fieldwork, including, importantly, all nine leaders.

Without the constraints of an academic programme and a research protocol, I engaged with this community on different terms; I directed my energy toward collaborative action co-developed with whoever came to meet me. It might also be notable that without an expense budget or an outcome oriented personal agenda, I no longer served food at my activities. Far fewer people came to meet, most consistently the "young men leaders," but the meetings that we had felt more natural.

It was only in hindsight that I realised the extent to which I had conceptualised participation, membership, and leadership differently in my return visit as compared to the thesis research. For the thesis, it felt important to me to approach a clearly defined group so that I could consider all of its members. This approach proved to be inconsistent with the group's pre-established nature. By contrast, upon my return, I allowed interest and availability to drive participation. The second strategy was far more comfortable; so much more comfortable that it was only in writing up this case that I actively asked myself how participation was systematically impacted by issues beyond interest and availability.

Each of the two approaches to leadership and membership has its advantages and its flaws; the juxtaposition of the two approaches makes these more apparent. Considering that disability is a contentious and evolving phenomenon, it was likely to the long-term benefit of my work to face challenges with categorical member-ship early; hopefully in a way that stimulates me to reconsider the issue repeatedly.

Commentary on Case 4.2

Meghna Guhathakurta

The striking points that come across in Cleaver's narratives are how he encounters the intersectional character of the research group and how it led him to innovate ways and methods of approach even outside the academic paradigm in which he initially found himself. PR groups are not usually expected to be monolithic in character. The PR methodology should in fact orient the researcher to deal with differences and diversities as much as looking at the collective whole. Intra-group tensions should also be taken in their stride. However, for all these differences and tensions to emerge progressively and to work through them, time and experience was needed, which are often not available to the academic. This is what the researcher realised and therefore went back to the group when the pressure of having to complete his research was not there.

The organic relationship he enjoyed with the same group, albeit a differently construed one, proved to be more fruitful as he says in his own words. 'Without an expense budget or an outcome oriented personal agenda, I no longer served food at my activities. Far fewer people came to meet, most consistently the "young men leaders", but the meetings that we had felt more natural.'

Case 4.3 Suicide and well-being: A participatory study with Inuit in Arctic Canada

Michael J. Kral

Introduction

This case is from a study on suicide and well-being among Inuit in Nunavut, Arctic Canada, funded by Health Canada. Like in the U.S., most Indigenous people in Canada live in urban areas. Most Inuit live in the Arctic in relatively small communities. Inuit constitute about 5 per cent of Indigenous people in Canada, totaling a little over 50,000 people according to the 2006 Canada census. They live in four regions, one of which, Nunavut, is a political territory since 1999. Evidence has been found that people lived there 4,000 years ago. While White people were involved with Inuit from missionaries to fur trading companies to police in the early twentieth century, the major colonial act was when the Canadian government took over their lives starting in the late 1950s. Inuit were moved from their family camps to crowded settlements, which are now their communities, their children were removed and sent to residential or day schools, and a wage economy was introduced which created poverty. At that time Inuit feared *Qallunaat* ('non-Inuit'). I have found that older Inuit believe their social problems began with the move into settlements.

The case

This is a case of power and privilege concerning gender, age, and ethnicity. I have always worked on research teams, and it is important that everyone gets along. Participatory research is supposed to remove hierarchies, emphasising reciprocity, democracy, respect, innovation, collaboration, the sharing of power, and is based on principles of community empowerment, ecology, social justice, feminism, and critical theory.

This study had Inuit research questions and the participatory method they wanted. It was the first time I had heard of participatory research, and I learned it from Inuit as an Indigenous research method. Working with two Inuit and two *Qallunaat* interviewers we interviewed 100 Inuit of all ages in two communities about well-being and happiness, sadness, health, culture change, and suicide.

There was an Inuit Steering Committee and academic researchers working closely together, and youth committees from each community were very involved, as well.

The research questions came from Inuit at a conference on suicide prevention. One of our interviewers, Padluq (a pseudonym) was a middle-aged Inuit man. At one point in the research we began to experience problems with Padluq. We would go on talk radio, where at lunch you can go on the radio and everybody in the community listens and can call in. This has become a tradition in Inuit communities. Padluq had recently finished rehab for drug addiction. When any of us went on the radio it was to talk about the research project, get input, etc. Whenever he went on the radio he would talk about his rehab and how he had been saved by Jesus. In his interviews he also talked a lot about rehab and Jesus rather than interviewing people. I had asked him to stop talking about this and to get on with the interviews, but he persisted. He had a negative attitude toward the youth we were working with, an Inuit youth committee that was very much involved in the project. They helped develop the interview questions. He also did not like working with women, specifically the two female interviewers, one White and one Inuit. He would complain about them when we met every morning to discuss the previous day's interviews.

The president of the Inuit youth committee finally came up to me and said that Padluq needs more counselling and should not be working with us. This was tough for me. As lead researcher I was now supposed to fire him. This made me feel bad, and I wondered about the ethics of doing this. A *Qallunaat* firing an Inuit. Race may be an issue. And it appears to go against participatory research, where power is supposed to be equal. This was an Indigenous person and I was half White (Roma; I look White and am a *Qallunaat*). I set up a meeting with Padluq, having prepared to tell him that other workers on the project were not getting along with him. Before I told him anything he said he was quitting because he was angry with a number of our collaborators, both Inuit and White (the White graduate student doing interviews). So we agreed that he would stop. He was also angry with me, saying that I was being paid more than the others. I was not getting any money at all from this grant. Our parting was difficult, and he said he was leaving because he did not want to listen to women and youth and that there was a 'White' problem.

After he left, as he was from another community, everything went well. But this was a tough thing to go through. I ran into him in his community several years later, and he was very friendly with me. I was relieved. This case made me think about what happens when a member of a research team does not get along with the others. Race, gender, and age can be important ethical issues, and here it was out in the open. I and the others, including the youth involved in the study, would not tolerate this. It was difficult to go through this process, but we were all glad after he left. This case raises issues about power, however, and the dynamics of race and gender. I and my Inuit partners were uncomfortable around this man, and they saw me as the person to do something about it.

Commentary on Case 4.3

Meghna Guhathakurta

PR engages pro-actively with power relations, both within and outside the group. But it is especially challenging if the researcher/s are located in a more powerful position in the social hierarchy than the participants themselves. This case illustrates the difficulties faced by the researcher in a graphic way.

Though the structure of the research was a collaborative one, it was precisely due to the differential social hierarchies that measures were taken to overcome the power imbalance between the Indigenous Inuit and White researchers, for example, there was an Inuit steering committee and academic research partners working together. The research questions came from Inuit at a conference on suicide prevention. Two Inuit and two *Qallunaat* were interviewers in two communities.

Despite this, challenges emerged at a personal level in the case of one Indigenous researcher. The predicament that Kral faced with this individual was not something that was insurmountable or even unexpected, yet it teaches us something important. We may be researching with communities that have their own structural boundaries, but they are communities that are also in transition and open to multiple influences of modernisation. This is where the dual trends of individuality and collectivity inherent in PR become useful. Individuals within a collective may have differences of opinion and trajectories, yet consider themselves as part of the whole. It is up to the 'outside' research institution to comprehend the nuances and prepare the researcher for such encounters and also engage the researcher in reflecting on his or her own positionality so that affective feelings like guilt and compassion may also be understood.

Case 4.4 Working with community conflict and ethnic tensions in a 'socially excluded locality' in the Czech Republic

Monika Bjeloncikova and Vendula Gojova

Introduction

This case has been written by two university researchers who were involved in community-based participatory research in an officially designated 'socially excluded locality' in the Czech Republic. According to the Czech government, a socially excluded locality is defined in terms of five forms of exclusion: spatial, social, economic, cultural and symbolic. A significant proportion of the residents of the locality were Roma people, and the researchers were keen to include them in the research. Roma people have been living in the Czech Republic for many generations, but the relations between ethnic majorities and minorities have been marred by the many ethnic prejudices that are constantly reinforced by the media. Roma people are spoken of as 'uneducated', 'uneducable', avoiding work and abusing the social system. These prejudices are reflected in urban housing policies, with Roma people frequently housed in locations which would be regarded as undesirable for most people. They also encounter discrimination in the employment market and education. The Czech Republic has been taken to the European Court of Human Rights to explain its approach to discriminatory practices on more than one occasion.

The case

The research took place in an urban area officially categorised as a 'socially excluded locality', which comprises a square, made up of low, brick-built blocks of flats, belonging to a private owner. The flats are in poor condition, occupied by about 800 people, mostly Roma or people on low incomes. People living in the houses in the neighbourhood immediately surrounding the area are mainly non-Roma people. Academics from the local university decided to initiate research on housing needs.

Some of the academics had participated in the implementation of community work in the area for over a year, resulting in the formation of a local group of 15 active citizens (of whom 12 were Roma people). We were in frequent contact with community workers operating in the locality during their work for a whole year before commencing our research. It became repeatedly apparent that the community workers worked with the local group on goals which were easily achievable in the short term, and for which they had sufficient information. The longer-term needs of the community were identified, including: a large playground; communication with the private owner of flats about the strategy for renting and maintaining the properties; and communication with the municipality about its plan for the socially excluded locality. However, these needs were assigned a lower priority, as to satisfy them would require work over a longer time period, based on more information to plan a strategy.

We adopted a participatory action research approach, anchored in the community – Community-Based Participatory Research. We assumed that the research could help the community in achieving their long-term goals, but we could see at the first meetings with representatives of active citizens from the locality and its surrounding neighbourhood (non-Roma people were interested in information about the research) that the people were very frustrated by their situation, and it would be difficult to free them from the stigma associated with generally negative perceptions of the people living in these so-called 'socially excluded locations' and the surrounding neighbourhoods. The situation was intensified by inter-ethnic tension (Roma people living in the flats versus those in the surrounding neighbourhood). Nevertheless, the fact that people came to the meeting and discussed their needs and problems (which were common for both 'sides') convinced us that these people definitely did not have a passive attitude towards their lives. A research working group was formed, comprising four Roma members from the socially excluded locality, four non-Roma people from the neighbourhood, and three academic researchers.

In the first two months of the research process, all the Roma members gradually left the research working group. They were residents of the locality, who were at the same time active in the existing local group and, sooner or later, all of them became overloaded by the activities of the two groups. There was also some ambiguity regarding the objectives and activities of the two groups. Nevertheless, during the mapping of the research field situation, and while searching for potential research topics at broader meetings with the residents of the larger administrative district, it was discovered that what plagued them and what they wanted to be changed was not connected with whether they were Roma or non-Roma people, whether they were residents of the so-called socially excluded locality, or even whether they were residents of the broader neighbourhood. Actually, they were all plagued by the quality of the housing environment, particularly: 1) dismal public space; 2) a lack of opportunities for leisure time; and 3) a rapid drop in the feeling of safety, which the residents of the administrative district associated with the influx of a large number of new residents into the socially excluded locality over the last year.

The research group participants chose to deal with the first two topics. However, to some extent, they were also addressed by the local group formed on the basis of community work.

We, as academic researchers, still had the idea in mind that research on the housing needs of residents of a socially excluded locality aimed to support the process of community work by supplying information 'about the people and their lives together with other people'. We perceived the concurrence of topics addressed by both groups as a confirmation that our idea of the research as a supporting tool of community work was exactly right. Yet the relations between the two groups, including the 'professional' members (community workers and academic research-ers), were rather tense. The research group was perceived more as competition than as providing assistance or support.

At the point when we were trying to understand the whole situation, an inter-national expert on community work was on a week-long visit to our university. We asked her for a consultation. With her and the community workers, we jointly considered issues that proved to be crucial for the activity of all active residents, considering the questions: what is the difference between the community work of the existing community workers, and the research work of the newly established research group, and what should their relationship be? The consultation helped to detect some causes of the tense situation, as follows:

- We, as academic researchers, had not devoted enough time to explaining the research as a support tool for existing community work to the community workers, members of the local group, and residents of the city district.
- One of the community workers (a Roma woman) pointed out that members of the local group were Roma people, and the research group members were non-Roma people. This may lead to concerns in the local group that the non-Roma people in the research group would 'roll over them', leading things in

their own direction, for their own benefit and to the disadvantage of Roma people.

It followed from the consultation that it was necessary to keep repeating to all those involved that the research group is a kind of information service for the local group, and that its activity serves to support the activities of the local group. As regards the difference in ethnicity and status (residents of the socially excluded locality vs. residents of the neighbourhood), we began to consider it an opportunity *to unite the people and empower them as residents of one administrative district*, forgotten and (in the citizens' words) 'thrown overboard' by the local municipality. From this perspective, we see participatory research as a way to achieve a higher degree of residents' participation, and to enhance social cohesion.

However, cooperation between the two groups remains marked by ethnic differences and the related burden of mutual prejudices: 'Non-Roma people just want to use our Roma people for their own benefit'; 'Around us, they pretend to be decent citizens, but amongst their own they behave like all the other Roma people'. This case highlights the ethnic tensions that are ever-present in localities and the potential for conflict, confusion, and disputes when university researchers attempt to engage with existing community workers and community groups.

Commentary on Case 4.4

Meghna Guhathakurta

This case illustrates similar problems to earlier cases where the researchers had to address a group that was already defined by local authorities as a socially excluded neighbourhood, where a mix of Roma and non-Roma people lived. Although the researchers tried to minimise the differences and tensions between the two groups in airing out problems that concerned both, it was challenging as the researchers, being university teachers, were thought to be higher up in the social hierarchy than the participants themselves. Gaining trust was therefore their first challenge. What was interesting in this particular case was that the researchers explicitly tried to explore the opportunities of bringing the group together ('*to unite the people and empower them as residents of one administrative district*') despite the differences and they skillfully practised their PR to that end. They however recorded the differences that remained within the group.

In community-based research, just as it is important to bring people together on a common agenda, it is also important to build the capacity of the group itself to see how the dynamics introduced to the group can be continued in the future to address the differences that remain. That may not be the objective of the authority or institution in question, in this case the local administration, but it definitely is within the agenda of PR pedagogy. It would be interesting to see how the civic engagement of universities could be continued and followed up in communities such as these for future learning purposes.

PART 3: CONCLUDING COMMENTS

Meghna Guhathakurta

As the cases and commentaries in this chapter illustrate, ethical issues are not simply add-ons to PR, but form part and parcel of the pedagogy itself. The preparation for such research must therefore form part of the curriculum of universities and other learning bodies. It must be a subject for discussion and reflection among individual researchers themselves, as well as mentors and supervisors. Universities and learning institutions should maintain continuous links with the communities and find creative ways in which community issues can find a space in the curriculum and classroom. Policy-makers of such institutions should also think of how to engage communities in decision-making and fund-raising for programmes that can mutually benefit each other (Brydon-Miller et al., 2006).

Conceptually, discussion of community rights, conflict and democratic representation in the context of ethics in participatory research leads us to interrogate these concepts, explore tensions that lie within and among them, and foreground spaces of a deepening understanding that can be co-created by diverse actors. Hopefully, such an understanding will in turn lead to transformative processes and pedagogies within institutions and in individual consciousness.

References

Barazangi, N. H. (2006). An ethical theory of action research pedagogy. *Action Research*, 4(1), 97–115.

Brydon-Miller, M., Greenwood, D., & Eikeland, O. (2006). Strategies for addressing ethical concerns in action research. *Action Research*, 4(1), 129–131.

Communities and Local Government Committee (2015). *Community Rights*. HC Report 262 https://publications.parliament.uk/pa/cm201415/cmselect/cmcomloc/262/26202.htm last accessed 30 November 2017.

Cooke, W. & Kothari, U. (2001). *Participation, the new tyranny*. London: Zed Books.

Donnelly, J. (1984). Cultural relativism and universal human rights. *Human Rights Quarterly*, 6(4), 400–419.

Gaventa, J. (1995). Citizen knowledge, citizen competence and democracy building. *The Good Society, 5(3), 28–35.*

Goldfarb, N. E. & Shamoo, A. E. (2008). Individual vs. community rights in clinical research. *Journal of Clinical Research Best Practices*, 4(10), https://firstclinical.com/journal/2008/0810_Rights.pdf last accessed 30 November 2017.

Guhathakurta, M. (forthcoming). University engagement in Bangladesh and its implication for alternative pedagogies. *CMU Journal.*

Louis, V. (2014). Concept Mapping. In D. Coghlan & M. Brydon-Miller (Eds.), *The SAGE encyclopedia of action research* (pp. 172–174). Los Angeles: SAGE Publications.

Lundy, P. & McGovern, M. (2006). The ethics of silence: Action research, community 'truth-telling' and post-conflict transition in the North of Ireland. *Action Research*, 4(1), 49–64.

Rahman, Md. A. (1994). *People's self-development, perspectives on participatory action research: A journey through experience*. London: Zed Books.

Rohmann, C. (1999). *A world of ideas: A dictionary of important theories, concepts, beliefs, and thinkers*. New York: Ballantine Publishing Group.

Rothman,J. (2014). Conflict management. In D. Coghlan & M. Brydon-Miller (Eds.), *The SAGE encyclopedia of action research* (pp. 174–175). Los Angeles: SAGE Publications.

Shemer, O. (2014). Community dialogue. In D. Coghlan & M. Brydon-Miller (Eds.), *The SAGE encyclopedia of action research* (pp. 143–146). Los Angeles: SAGE Publications.

Stoecker, R. (2014). Community development. In D. Coghlan & M. Brydon-Miller (Eds.), *The SAGE encyclopedia of action research* (pp. 139–143). Los Angeles: SAGE Publications.

Vasilache, A. (2009). Cultural Relativism and Human Rights, In A. Petchsiri, J. L. D. Marques, & W. Roth (Eds.), *Promoting human rights in Asia and Europe* (pp. 43–57). Downloaded from https://www.nomos-elibrary.de/10.5771/9783845220321-43/cultural-relativism-and-human rights, last accessed 30 November 2017.

Ward, L. F. (1909). Ludwig Gumplowicz. *American Journal of Sociology, 12*(3), 410–413.

Ward, L. F. & Gumplowicz, L. (1971). *The Ward-Gumplowicz correspondence: 1897–1909*. Oakland, CA: Essay Press.

5

CO-OWNERSHIP, DISSEMINATION AND IMPACT

Gustaaf Bos and Tineke Abma

With cases contributed by Kate York, Sarah Marie Wiebe, Aila-Leena Matthies, Gustaaf Bos and Rafaella Van Den Bosch, and additional commentaries by Truus Teunissen and Doortje Kal

PART 1: INTRODUCTION AND OVERVIEW OF THE ISSUES

Gustaaf Bos and Tineke Abma

Background

The term 'co-ownership' is recently emerging in the research fields of health care and social well-being. The notion is ill-defined, but a key idea is that when people co-create knowledge, as in participatory research (PR), they should also equally share and own this knowledge and accompanying innovations. The reason for interest in co-ownership is the increasing acceptance that not only academics have the right or capability to inquire about the world in which we live. This relates to redressing the balance of power and interests, and one of the most prominent ethical issues in sharing control and co-ownership throughout the research process is how to prevent the colonisation, co-option and appropriation of the voices and stories of less powerful people by vested interests. This 'taking over' is not always intended, but nevertheless may be felt as such because it re-establishes structural inequalities in the research field – a topic we discuss later in the chapter.

Dissemination and impact are related topics that refer to sharing research findings and the influence of research on the lives of people concerned. In PR, pathways to dissemination and impact are characterised by a participatory ethics and spirit. That is, dissemination and impact are key to the whole enterprise; change and action for change are the driving forces (see Abma et al., 2018; also Chapter 7 in this volume). Moreover, dissemination and impact are not solely controlled by academics, but shared with research partners. Jointly it is decided what should be disseminated to whom and what impact is desirable. Ethical issues relate to prioritising audiences, representations and agency, as well as who decides what counts as beneficial impact.

This chapter discusses ethical issues that may arise in striving towards co-ownership, participatory dissemination and impact. Following a systematic literature search, we conclude that this topic appears not to be extensively discussed. In Part 1 we offer an overview of some of the main issues raised in the available literature. Then four cases from different places around the world are presented in Part 2: Tanzania, Canada, Finland, and the Netherlands. The cases discuss ethical challenges within different contexts, including rural African villages, a Canadian First Nation community and two European urbanised areas, involving research with people with access to a medication distribution programme, Indigenous people, unemployed young men, and people with intellectual disabilities.

Together with Truus Teunissen and Doortje Kal, who identify themselves as activists, we (Gustaaf Bos and Tineke Abma) comment on each case briefly, drawing on our experiences. All four of us are white Dutch and have worked together in PR projects for some years. Truus has multiple chronic diseases, and has written counter-stories and auto-ethnographies based on her personal experiences (Teunissen et al., 2013). Once a prevention worker in the field of social psychiatry, Doortje is the 'godmother' of the 'Kwartiermaken' approach, which aims for more societal space for people with psychiatric and intellectual disabilities and other marginalised groups (Kal, 2001; 2012). Gustaaf and Tineke work from the academy. Gustaaf is a post-doctoral researcher at VU university, Amsterdam, working on the topic of personal encounters between people from the margins and people from mainstream society (Bos, 2016; Bos & Kal, 2016). Tineke is Professor of Participation and Diversity at VU, and has written extensively on responsive evaluation and PR approaches (Abma et al., 2009).

Understanding co-ownership

The notion of co-ownership emerged in a context in which voices of service users (this term includes 'clients' and 'patients'), families and advocacy groups are increasingly considered relevant, valid and complementary to perspectives of professionals and academic researchers. Besides substantive and pragmatic considerations (it leads to better care, better implementation), normative arguments lie at the core of this development. The choice to involve service users is supported by value-laden arguments: they have a right to be involved because they are the end-users, and are thus considered stakeholders in research. Their perspectives and experiential knowledge can contribute to the research process, and lead to research that better relates to the needs and expectations of service users (Entwistle et al., 1998; Faulkner & Thomas, 2002; Staniszewska et al., 2007). Arnstein's (1969) participation ladder illustrates different levels at which citizens gain increasing control or decision-making power in policy and practice. In health research, this ladder has been adapted to encompass degrees of service user (patient) involvement (Abma et al., 2009). Three levels of participation can be distinguished, which are relevant to better understand the notion of co-ownership: consultation, control and collaboration.

Consultation is one of the commonest strategies for inclusion. This strategy involves people as information-givers or advisors. Examples include nominating research topics (Caron-Flinterman et al., 2005; www.lindalliance.org/index.asp), and consulting service users on designing clinical trials (Marsden & Bradburn, 2004). It also includes incorporating into the research the views and experiences of people in under-represented groups, often marginalised and regarded by outsiders as 'vulnerable', for example, older people and people with intellectual disabilities or mental health problems (Knox et al., 2000; Hellstrom et al., 2007; McVilly et al., 2006; Richardson, 2000). However, decision-making power still stays with the researchers.

Control means that people whose lives are the subject of the study, for example, service users, relatives or advocacy groups, have primary decision-making power over all strategic choices in research. Examples include studies where service users help to formulate a research bid and decide on the research and methodologies (Buckley et al., 2007; Staniszewska et al., 2007) or act as entrepreneurs, for example in the Duchenne parent project (www.duchenne.nl) and PXE International (www.pxe.org). User-led or survivor-led research, developing in the field of psychiatry and Mad Studies, can also be categorised under the control model (Russo & Beresford, 2015; Rose, 2017). The power clearly shifts to the service users and survivors being in control (versus academic researchers) in a response to the domination and silencing of mad voices: '*balancing* the overwhelming majority of material written about those who are labelled mad by those who do the labelling and those who study them' (Kalathil & Crepaz-Keay, 2013, in: Russo & Beresford, 2015, p. 153).

Although consultation and control differ in degrees of participation, in both instances one party leads the interaction. Either professional researchers are in charge by formulating questions to which service users and families can respond (consultation), or relatives, users and survivors are in charge by determining the research (control). This is not to say that iterative contacts between service users/families/survivors and researchers do not exist. There are situations where service users control some research, and engage with researchers who conduct the work, under guidance of the service users. The point is that power and ownership lie in the hands of one actor and dialogue and interaction are minimised.

Collaboration is quite different, with service users as 'co-researchers' involved in all stages of the research process, sharing control and co-labouring on an equal basis with academic researchers in an ongoing process of dialogue and interaction. It should be noted that this is a prescriptive definition and an ideal. Striving towards equality is one matter, but realising it in practice is much more difficult and always requires an alertness about power differentials and how these play out. In a context where professional researchers have always been the dominant and established parties, and thus might take their privileged position for granted, a special sensitivity to use and misuse of power is required. There are few empirical studies describing this degree of participation. Examples include studies on migraine (Belam et al.,

2005), intellectual disabilities (Abell et al., 2007; Nierse & Abma, 2011), schizo-phrenia (Schneider et al., 2004) and former sex workers (Benoit et al., 2005).

Collaboration entails sharing power and promoting co-ownership among pro-fessional researchers and those whose lives or work are at stake. The aim of the next section is to examine ethical issues that emerge around co-ownership. This differs from legal or managerial approaches to co-ownership, such as those found in the literature on intellectual property and co-patenting in business partnerships (Belderbos et al., 2014).

Ethical issues related to co-ownership of research

We now discuss ethical issues relating to the dangers of apparently co-owned research turning into either 1) colonisation, or 2) co-option of the ideas, expe-riences and opinions of community-based researchers by professional researchers.

1. When co-ownership becomes colonisation

Russo and Beresford (2015, pp. 155–156) are critical about including service users' narratives in research and sharing of ownership:

> If the first problem was getting any kind of recognition for such narratives, then now this has begun to be achieved it appears we may have moved on to a further stage when an additional issue emerges. This is how to ensure that they are not just colonized or reduced to a new area for academic activity – taken from the control of their own authors.

These authors point out that the intention of co-ownership may turn into a dis-appointing experience when people's narratives and voices are 'taken over' for interpretation and analysis by academics reframing and taking the experiences from them. The concept of 'epistemic injustice' (Fricker, 2007) is relevant here, referring to the fact that not everyone is considered an authoritative knower. People with emotional instabilities or cognitive impairments are particularly at risk of being seen as lacking credibility as knowers (Fricker, 2007). Epistemic injustice includes testimonial injustice (a speaker is not regarded as credible by listeners) and herme-neutic injustice (a speaker does not have access to collectively valued interpretative resources to make sense of their own or others' experiences). According to Russo and Beresford (2015) even when there is testimonial justice (people dare to tell their stories), epistemic injustice continues through hermeneutic injustice (experts inter-preting the stories). The underlying dualism and opposition between experiences of people 'out there' and the inner realm of academia where these experiences are interpreted is repeated and a hierarchy deepened, because now a professional/ academic not only has the power to speak with academic authority, but also with reference to experiential knowledge. This is a situation called 'epistemic violence' (Boumans, 2012). What does it mean to work towards epistemic justice in equal partnership? This question remains largely unanswered. The first thing is recognising the power asymmetries (the privileged position of academic researchers in relation to the weak position of service users) that are always at stake, even when intentions are good. It points to the importance of reflexivity throughout the process (see Case 5.4).

2. When co-ownership becomes co-option

Involvement and co-ownership can become co-option. Co-option entails less powerful people being used in/for the agenda of professionals, academic researchers or policy-makers, ultimately reinforcing the status quo. This has been put on the agenda by various scholars, such as Turner & Gillard (2012) and Beresford & Russo (2016). In order prevent co-option, Beresford and Russo suggest we might learn from the field of Disability Studies. This enabled people with disabilities to understand their disabilities as caused by deficiencies in social environments rather than impairments of their minds or bodies. This helped people with disabilities to reframe their lives, undo oppression and internalisation of oppression. Oliver (2013, p. 1025, in Beresford and Russo, 2016, p. 272), who introduced the social model of disability in the 1980s, reflects critically:

> Many academic papers and some books have been published whose main concern has been to attack, reform or revise the social model, and reputations and careers have been built on the back of these attacks.

Oliver suggests that the intellectual debate on the social model has been rich and beneficial for academia, but not much has changed for people with disabilities. In short, who benefits from the work generated by the people with disabilities? Who owns it? (See Case 5.2.)

Understanding dissemination

In PR projects, 'dissemination' (sharing knowledge with others) is a multi-layered phenomenon. Authors on this topic may refer to dissemination as an essential and integrated feature of PR, as well as a phase and a consequence of their research (Abma et al., 2019; Banks et al., 2013; Quigley, 2006; Wilson et al., 2018). Seen as a *characteristic* feature of PR, dissemination is based on a conviction that if academics wish to contribute to improving the lives of people who are often marginalised, they should ensure equal access to, and a mandate in, every phase of the research process (Abma et al., 2019; Banks et al., 2013). Next to this, dissemination is defined as a distinct research *phase*, occurring right after the writing up of research results and insights, and embodied, for example, as documentary films, photos, dialogue sessions or symposia, academic articles, leaflets and easy read publications (Abma et al., 2019; Wilson et al., 2018). Dissemination is also conceived of as a broader (and longer lasting) research *consequence*, meant to 'engender change, to engage [other] people in further critical reflection, dialogue, learning, imagination and action' with regards to the topic a stake (Abma et al., 2019, Chapter 9). Consequently, instead of being narrowly defined, the concept of dissemination rather encapsulates a variety of ways in which PR facilitates the proliferation of knowledge that is assembled throughout collaborative processes of knowledge sharing and meaning-making.

Ethical issues related to dissemination

Issues about dissemination are often intertwined with concerns regarding the impact of research and co-ownership of results (Bromley et al., 2015; Cordner et al., 2012 in Wilson et al., 2018). Some of the most crucial ethical questions regarding dissemination are: Who decides what should be disseminated, to whom, and in what ways? Who takes responsibility and leadership? Which are the main priority groups and how to reach them? How do we deal with discriminatory or stigmatising public images of the people and contexts that are the subject of the study?

In the following section, we discuss these issues:

1. Responsibility and leadership.
2. Prioritising and reaching audience groups.
3. Representation.

1. Responsibility and leadership

In disseminating collaboratively produced knowledge, ideally decisions about responsibilities and leadership should be discussed and planned by all research team members. Jointly the team can decide who will be involved, who is responsible and who does what. If, for example, academic publications are considered relevant then academics might take the lead. In other instances community partners and/or service users might be more appropriate leaders in dissemination.

In attempting to tackle issues of leadership in advance, some participatory projects discuss and develop (written) agreements about dissemination procedures (Banks et al., 2013; Gilchrist, 2015; Quigley, 2006). Such formal contracts, or less formal working agreements, are useful to gain some clarity over responsibilities.

2. Prioritising and reaching audience groups

PR always produces knowledge for a variety of stakeholder groups, for example, the people involved, the general public, other academics, advocacy groups, support or health care professionals. When the PR team discusses disseminating their results, they might encounter disagreement about which group should go first. Case 5.2, about dissemination of a documentary film co-produced by Indigenous young people and a doctoral researcher, offers an example.

Another issue relates to the use of appropriate language and media to reach various audiences. Using academic jargon might help get a message across in academic contexts, whilst being alienating and obstructive in many other situations, for example when informing patients or service users about clinical guidelines (Coulter & Ellins, 2007; Eccles et al., 2012). In the latter case, it is recommended to make dissemination plans at an early stage and involve service users throughout the process, including in the translation of jargon into lay language (Schipper et al., 2016).

Another device is using 'plain language' (Durham Community Research Team, 2011) designed for all audiences to understand, versus communicating in different 'styles' and 'grammars' for specific groups. Plain language (written or performative) might indeed facilitate a more democratic and heterogenous dialogue about issues of social (in)equality and (in)justice between people from the margins and the mainstream of a social system. Hence the use of plain language may endorse reciprocal processes of meaning-making. However, plain language might also deny important nuances that help some audiences to think thoroughly about the issue at stake. Consequently, the approach to this issue might unjustly appear too linear. Such simplification might not only hinder further ethical deliberation between everyone involved, but also weaken the motivation to keep searching for good ways to respond to the perspectives of other stakeholders, even when these responses might never be fully adequate (Bos & Kal, 2016).

Therefore, the challenge is how our sharing of PR insights can deconstruct and 'mess about' divisive boundaries, expectations, partnerships, structures and routines, without oversimplifying their influence in everyday life and ignoring essential (interpersonal and contextual) differences between the members of our audiences.

3. Representation

Representation refers to how people and their life worlds are depicted and disclosed to others. Important issues include use of jargon and professional categories. Should any medically, socially and/or culturally charged labels be used to describe those involved or are these labels deliberately not used to prevent stigmatisation? If it is unclear whether non-academic researchers are able to decide for themselves how they want to be represented, for example due to cognitive limitations, the concept of 'relational agency' (Burkitt, 2015; Waldenfels, 2004) applies. Concretely, this means that people need to be supported in their decisions about how they are depicted.

When portraying life world contexts, the notion of 'place-based stigma' is helpful. It refers to the disgust and vilification applied to geographical areas that suffer economically and socially (Byrne et al., 2015). Media can play an important role in reproducing images of, for example, 'bad' or 'dangerous' neighbourhoods. Whether accurate or not, these images have an impact on residents. Members of the research team need to make choices in this respect, and to anticipate and account for harmful dynamics despite their good intentions (Brabeck et al., 2015; Brugge & Cole, 2003; Walsh et al., 2008; cf. Abma et al., 2019, Chapter 9).

Understanding impact

Through shared meaning-making processes, PR strives towards social justice and change (Banks et al., 2013; Banks et al., 2017), and has always been focused on 'impact' in the broad sense – understood as the cultural, social or economic influence of the research project beyond the academic context.

Over the last two decades, demand from funding bodies to demonstrate the societal impact of any research project has increased (Banks et al., 2017). In response to this, community and PR approaches have begun to describe the wider social impact of their work (Cook & Roche, 2017), arguing that impact occurs throughout the PR process (not only at the end after the findings are produced), and everyone involved decides on what impact should be realised (Abma et al., 2019).

Pathways to impact are not linear and often 'messy' (Cook, 2009), because although impact may be tangible and concrete in some instances (e.g. practical, political and structural changes/decisions), more often it is intangible, diffuse and porous (e.g. heightened individual and/or shared understandings, new conceptualisations, see Pain et al., 2015). Similarly, impact may happen instantly – during or directly after the research ends – but also more gradually and over long periods of time (i.e. through a ripple effect).

Ethical issues related to impact

PR team members share motivations to stimulate more social equality and justice among the people concerned. Consequently, this emancipatory stance is an important catalyst for the type of impact the research team wants to achieve.

At the same time, representatives of varying stakeholder groups may also have diverging motives, priorities and positions in relation to the central research theme, as seen in Case 5.1, which discusses disagreements between research partners in Tanzania about when and how to disseminate findings. Similarly, different stakeholders might also appreciate results differently and/or may strive for different, sometimes even conflicting, outcomes (Banks et al., 2017).

Besides, a PR project may yield unexpected, involuntary, and even unpleasant, outcomes for some participants. Hence, ethical issues concerning the expected and unexpected impact of PR inevitably touch upon the question of to what extent the research team and its individual members can influence what their shared project generates and stimulates, and how they can be held accountable for unforeseen negative consequences.

Next we discuss some everyday ethical issues around the impact of PR, covering:

1. Selecting and prioritising research outcomes.
2. Impact of the research process and outcomes on participants.
3. Who determines what is (most) beneficial?

1. Selecting and prioritising research outcomes

PR approaches aim to be beneficial for all participants, but especially for the most marginalised people involved. This presupposes that throughout the process, team members share an awareness about what is beneficial for each of them. Therefore, PR teams should keep discussing members' expectations and experiences related to the research outcomes throughout the research process.

Furthermore, the research team has to enable all research participants to relate to the research outcomes in ways that suit them. In other words, the people involved need to be supported by the research team to apply research insights and outcomes constructively to their life worlds, in order to facilitate desired changes – what Guba and Lincoln (1989) call 'tactical authenticity'. This requires insight into which 'capabilities' (e.g. skills, knowledge, network membership, see Nussbaum, 2006) each research participant needs to profit from the research process and results (Walsh et al., 2008).

Another question is whether the applicability and value of the research outcomes should be considered in a concrete or an abstract sense. Are the people involved satisfied if the analysis of the university researcher identifies intangible changes, e.g. more 'relational empowerment' (Baur et al., 2010) or enlarged mutual understanding, or do they demand a more measurable transformation, such as written commitment from policy-makers, positive media exposure or broad public interest in their research product (see Case 5.1 about health research in Tanzania)?

Similarly, what selection criteria are used to determine results most suitable for publication? What happens when results relevant to current policy and/or scientific discourses and results relevant to the people involved are different, or even contradictory? These questions have to be handled when the research team selects and prioritises research outcomes.

2. Impact of research processes and outcomes on participants

Authors writing about research impact state that both the research process (Greene, 2013; Mistry et al., 2015 in Wilson et al., 2018) and research results (Mitchell & Baker, 2005; Williams et al., 2010) may have desired and undesired impact on people's lives. This is often hard to indicate or influence.

Frequently, issues of privacy and confidentiality are at stake, which are especially hard to overcome since community researchers often owe their very position to disclosure of parts of their personal lives and experiences (Banks et al., 2013; Wilson et al., 2018). Sharing their stories in (often small-scale) participatory projects might endanger intra community relationships (Williams et al., 2010) as well as broader societal bonds. Expressing minority viewpoints or disclosing activity might result in economic deprivation (Walsh et al., 2008), prosecution or stigmatisation (Brabeck et al., 2015; Teti et al., 2012; Vishalache & Cornforth, 2013) or unwanted responses from policy-makers (Rink et al., 2013). The issue here is how we should anticipate and respond in an adequate way to these 'impact risks'.

Apart from these undesirable consequences, some PR projects are confronted with an apparent lack of impact: nothing seems to happen as a result of their efforts (see Case 5.3, about the lack of policy change in response to young people's recommendations). The underlying problem here might be that many participatory projects aim to facilitate local action based on situational, temporal and relational knowledge, whereas policy-makers tend to appreciate and focus on aggregated and generalisable research findings. Hence, the change each party strives for is different in character and scope: organic and small-scale versus structured and large-scale. In order to deal with this tension, the PR team should facilitate ongoing dialogue between the stakeholder groups about expectations, issues and concerns throughout the research process.

3. Who determines what is (the most) beneficial impact?

When it comes to determining which impact is beneficial, a PR team might need to address the worldviews, beliefs, values and norms of its members and other stakeholder groups. Which (moral) principles and (idealistic) notions are applied to decide preferred changes? Who has the final say in this decision-making process?

Again, the question of short-term versus long-term is relevant. Quite often (participatory) research attempts to change something for the short term, because funding for working on longer-term transformation is hard to get. Related to this is the tendency of policy-makers and funding bodies to demand quantitative, measurable results, although invisible transformations – e.g. deepened mutual insight and understanding – might be more profound and decisive (Abma et al., 2019, Chapter 10).

PART 2: CASES AND COMMENTARIES

Case 5.1 Disagreements about ownership of data and use of findings: Ethical issues in community-based health research in Tanzania

Kate York

Introduction

This case is written by a qualified nurse from the USA, undertaking research as a PhD student on a community-based research project in Tandai, a village in the Morogoro Rural Region of Tanzania. The area is the breeding ground for the black fly that carries the parasitic worm onchocerca volvulus. Tandai is one of over 5,000 villages in Tanzania where onchocerciasis, the disease caused by the parasite, is endemic. This leads to insufferable itching, skin lesions, and sometimes, blindness. There is a yearly medication distribution programme aimed at eventual eradication of the disease by a sustained 15-year treatment/prevention programme. The programme is managed through the Ministry of Health, an international non governmental development organisation (NGDO), and regional and local staff from affected districts in Tanzania. This community-based research project was a collaborative effort with the Tanzania Ministry of Health, Sightsavers International (SSI), Morogoro District Medical Officer, local directors of the African Programme for Onchocerciasis Control, and leaders and community members of Tandai and Kazinga villages.

The case

The sustainability of this programme was the focus of the community-based research project. Specifically, we were looking at factors affecting community members' participation in the yearly programme and the role of community health workers. There were two issues within this collaboration that were challenging. First, we worked with key stakeholders in the programme and collaborated with local programme coordinators and village leaders for survey data collection, key informant interviews and focus group discussions (FGDs). The NGDO provided access to transportation, driver, programme coordinators, and local people who would participate as part of the research team. We planned for four FGDs: one for women who participated in the programme, one for men who participated; and one for women and one for men who didn't participate.

On the morning of the FGDs, all the community members who agreed to participate were waiting outside the school building we would be using. Being a fledgling researcher in a foreign country, I hadn't anticipated this issue. We only had one FGD facilitator and me to conduct the FGDs. We had agreed to stagger the times, but this hadn't happened. The leaders assured me the participants wouldn't mind waiting. The first two groups had participated in the medication distribution programme. The FGDs went well and participants seemed happy. The third group was the first of the male participants who didn't participate in the pro-gramme. There was a distinctly different attitude among these participants – slightly defensive and hostile.

At the end of the session, the participants refused to leave without payment for their time. There was no promise of payment, at least I hadn't mentioned payment when the research team met to go over the protocol. Protocols at both the Institutional Review Board (IRB) at my university and the National Institute of Medical Research were approved without incentives for participants, as I thought people would feel that it was part of the responsibility of a community member to better the health of the overall population. The group sat for a long time, but I was stubborn. I didn't have money to give them, nor was it part of the protocols. My focus group facilitator and the programme coordinator urged me to give in. But I held firm that we would need to sit all day, as I didn't have anything to give. Once this group finally left without payment, the last group of the day was to be women who didn't participate in the programme. We found they had gone home, having heard there was no monetary incentive for participating. I was willing to forgo the final FGD since those randomly chosen were no longer available. We left that village and had better luck with the next village, where we conducted the four sessions without incident.

However, my partner organisation was not willing to go without that missing focus group. They wanted to return for the opinions of the missing group. I was disappointed that we didn't have all four groups from the first village, but wrote it off as a learning experience. They agreed to pay for the driver, car and facilitator if I would try again. The programme coordinator telephoned the village leaders, who said they would have participants ready, but I would have to pay them. I said we couldn't pay as it wasn't in the protocol and the other participants weren't paid. They insisted. I tried to cancel the trip. I chatted with the village leader, clearly stating we would not be coming after all. He spoke to the coordinator and suddenly everything was fine and we were on our way. I was sceptical. We drove to the programme director's house; he handed money to the coordinator. I asked if this was for the participants, and he assured me it was not, but my gut told me differently. Off we went across the mountain.

We began the focus group and right away I felt this group was very different from the others comprising non-participants in the programme. Typically, participants were somewhat defensive and suspicious. These women were smiling, saying had they known the importance of the programme, they would of course have participated. When discussions concluded, we had an impromptu photo opportunity and everyone was cheery. I walked back to the room to grab my bag and witnessed the women being handed money. They were being paid for their participation, which likely influenced their responses, making the results of that group void. I contacted the Institutional Review Board, and they confirmed that we shouldn't use the data. The partnering organisation didn't see it this way. They wanted to use the data to report to the Ministry of Health. I didn't give in to their argument that they paid for that session and should have the results. The programme coordinator didn't understand the implications of his actions: that paying the participants negated the results. His intention was not to sabotage, but to help us get the groups we wanted in order to answer our questions. In the end, the data weren't used.

The second challenge was the dissemination of findings. I felt the villagers should have a chance to hear the results first and corroborate or disagree, so we could have the most accurate representation of the issues. Again, the NGDO had a different priority, which was to inform the Ministry of Health of preliminary findings in order to fit within the window of the next strategic planning cycle. At this point in the research, there was no more funding to go back to the villages for this important interaction, so preliminary findings were given to the Ministry of Health and I headed back to the USA, feeling like the research was incomplete. Dissemination of findings to the community was discussed prior to the start of the research, but when it was time to take data back to the villages, there was no cooperation from the partners. In the end, I returned a year later with the collaboration of the NGDO to disseminate the final report and discuss the recommendations. Thankfully, the reported findings were on target with the feedback from the community and I left with a sense that the work had a positive influence at the policy level and would eventually benefit the collaborating villages.

Commentary on Case 5.1

Tineke Abma, Truus Teunissen, Doortje Kal and Gustaaf Bos

In this case the researcher wrestled with the moral dilemma of whether or not to accede to demands to pay participants in two focus groups, although participants in other groups were not paid and payment was not agreed in the study protocol approved by the review board at her university in the USA. Although her local research collaborators requested that payment should be made, she held on to her principle. Later, however, participants in one focus group were paid behind her back by the partner organisation. The researcher felt the payment might have led participants to give socially desirable answers, and therefore the findings were not trustworthy.

We wonder if the socio-economic position of participants in this particular focus group (as well as the other groups) might have been such that paying them for their participation could be justified in this situation. We are reminded of Gilligan's (1982) argument from a care ethical perspective that particular circumstances might lead to action which is legally not allowed, but morally legitimated, because it nurtures and fosters the well-being of those under pressure. Might it have been reasonable to pay people for their involvement in the last focus group of the day, in this case because they waited a very long time before they could participate? We guess the answer depends on the particularities of the situation, such as the different socio-economic positions of the participants and the researcher (and representatives from other institutions). It might be argued that in future situations, in order to anticipate possible undesirable impact that could be linked to the vast socio-economic differentials between participants and researchers, all participants should get a certain reimbursement. Related to this is the dilemma about whether information to be gained from a focus group is worth the effort of a group of people waiting for hours before they can participate.

Another dilemma is that the researcher felt she needed to discuss the findings with the local community before disseminating them to policy-makers, but had no control over this process. Sharing findings first with the locals seems indeed preferable as argued in Part 1 of this chapter, because they are the primary 'owners' of the findings.

Case 5.2 Decolonising research through documentary film? Indigenous environmental justice and community-engagement in Canada

Sarah Marie Wiebe

Introduction

Written by an academic of non-Indigenous heritage, this case discusses ethical dilemmas faced while completing PhD fieldwork in an Indigenous community in Canada. In Canada there are over 600 First Nation communities. Some live on reserve lands whose treaty rights pre-date Canadian confederation in 1867. Others live on often marginalised land allocated by the federal government through patch-work policy decisions. No reserve or First Nations community is alike across the country. In 1982, the amended Canadian Constitution recognised and affirmed Aboriginal rights. The term 'Aboriginal' encompasses First Nations, Inuit and Métis peoples. Rather than use the legal term 'Aboriginal', many communities, activists and scholars prefer the term 'Indigenous'. As such, this case example uses this term in referring to these communities, their struggles for justice and the ongoing legacy of Canadian colonialism affecting Indigenous bodies, homes and lands today.

The case

After viewing a documentary film, *The Disappearing Male*, guided by community protocols and relationships as well as my intuition and passion for social justice, as a doctoral candidate, during the winter of 2011, I relocated from Ottawa – Canada's capital – to Aamjiwnaang, an Indigenous territory encircled by a noxious zone known as 'Chemical Valley'. This relocation coincided with my involvement on a collaborative research project focused on youth leadership and environmental awareness between the Aamjiwnaang First Nation Health and Environment Committee and York University, Toronto. As a Research Assistant on this project, working alongside academic researchers and community-members, I began to build relationships within the community. I soon relocated and continued to support youth leadership on a voluntary basis while commencing my own research on environmental and reproductive justice due to Canada's colonial toxic body politics.

With a background in Political Science, my intention was to move beyond the formal institutional realm of politics in an attempt to come to grips with the lived realities for Indigenous citizens fighting for environmental and reproductive justice with their bodies on the frontlines of repeated pollution exposure. Surrounded by industry, this community confronts contamination on all fronts: in the air, soil and water, ultimately, impacting their home and penetrating their bodies. In 2005, a team of collaborative researchers produced a study revealing that the number of male births drastically decreased. I soon learned that the skewed birth ratio was but one concern in Aamjiwnaang among many. Cancer, asthma and cardiovascular illnesses affect nearly each family and home, coupled by fear of the everyday landscape. With the repeated sounds of chemical alert sirens, felt vibrations from neighbouring smokestacks and bittersweet smell of unknown substances, which one can almost taste when driving south from the City of Sarnia along Vidal Road onto the Aamjiwnaang reserve, this is a deeply affective atmosphere.

Working with/in Indigenous communities requires recognition that these communities are some of the most 'researched' in the world. Drawing upon principles of respect, reciprocity and relationship-building, which are central to the Native Women's Association of Canada's vision of decolonising methodologies, I worked closely with a team of advisors including an Elder and maintained ongoing accountability to the Aamjiwnaang First Nation Health and Environment Committee. My research design involved community-situated experts throughout all phases including the proposal, development of recruitment materials, operations and dissemination of findings. While living in Aamjiwnaang territory, I too connected to municipal emergency alert systems via cell phone and internet notifications, also heard the incessant sirens wail and shared real-time news updates through social media. During my immersion in the field, I joined community activists with public speaking engagements and co-authored Letters to the Editor for the local paper. From this participatory-action approach, my intention was to share my privilege, voice and authority with the community to the best of my ability. Trying to move beyond an extractive form of knowledge production, I sought to work with and alongside the community with the shared pursuit of seeking justice and sharing knowledge.

During the final phase of my fieldwork, as I was gearing up to relocate back to Ottawa, youth leaders approached me with the request to work on a cross-cultural collaborative education project together in the local high school. After a series of brainstorming meetings including representatives from several youth groups based in the community, we came up with the collective vision of co-producing a documentary film. The Kiijig Collective was born and I stayed eight months longer than initially anticipated, bringing my field immersion close to two years. The cross-cultural collective brought together Indigenous and non-Indigenous youth with the aim of using creative means to speak up and out about injustices, stereotypes and environmental concerns. Our collective set out to screen the film at the local high school attended by the involved youth the following spring. Our group met at least weekly to discuss roles and responsibilities, schedule interviews and secure funding. As a researcher familiar with how to leverage various funding sources, the collective nominated me to take on the role of 'Executive Producer'. In this role, I oversaw the film's financing, and also assumed the role of 'Line Producer' and saw to it that our collective made it to scheduled meetings and interviews. Upon reflection, there are several ethical dilemmas that emerged out of this grassroots, youth-based and community-driven undertaking: the challenges of consensus-based decision-making, ownership and sustainability.

As mentioned, the Kiijig Collective formed out of a youth-led initiative to share knowledge about Indigenous values and beliefs with a non-Indigenous audience. We began with weekly meetings, inclusive to any Indigenous youth from Aamjiwnaang as well as non-Indigenous youth from the high school. Given the reality that young people have multiple priorities and interests competing for attention, we had about three to five members show up to meetings on a regular basis. Thus, this group became the de facto decision-makers. At times, when other members turned up, feelings of exclusion emerged and as a result, we repeatedly revisited our agenda, objectives and governing structure. This was one difficulty with consensus-based decision-making.

Second, the technical issue of 'ownership' made output a challenge. As a collaborative collective, we all agreed that no one member 'owned' the film. While we reached our goal of screening the film the following spring at the local high school, as well as at a few local conferences and one national festival, I felt that it would be inappropriate to speak as a hierarchical 'Executive Producer' on behalf of the film and stepped aside. Without consensus amongst the youth on the future vision for the film, I felt that it would be inappropriate for me to assume a key role as spokesperson for this project, although I was and continue to be very invested in the initiative. The film (publicly available on YouTube) has primarily been screened in an academic setting as a teaching tool for students and scholars. Only on a rare occasion when involved youth could not attend official screenings did I show up to speak on behalf of the collective at a film festival. At the time of my physical departure from the community in the fall of 2012, the youth were undecided on the film's next steps. As such, I've opted to respect their leadership and await direction on how best to disseminate the film.

Third and finally, given the transition from PhD candidate to academic employment, I've since relocated from the field, which raises the issue of project sustainability. My presence was a double-edged sword in many respects. On the one hand, it provided continuity to the project; on the other, it perhaps cramped out the capacity for the youth to speak out and shine themselves. Thus, issues of consensus, ownership and sustainability remain open questions, leaving the future of the film in limbo.

All said and done, working collaboratively in this setting proved to be an enriching and eye-opening initiative. Since leaving the field, I've kept in contact with community-members and continue to return to the community periodically to participate in community events whenever possible. For instance, in the fall of 2016, I launched my book *Everyday Exposure: Indigenous Mobilization and Environmental Justice in Canada's Chemical Valley in Sarnia* during a 'First Fridays' artist event in the downtown core with many community-members present to share their knowledge with the wider public. Despite the aforementioned challenges, I'm eternally grateful to the community for the numerous laughs and lessons learned. While I might do some things differently next time, I'm looking forward to working with this community and others on future innovative cross-cultural and mixed media storytelling projects down the road to interrupt colonial toxic body politics and collectively envision alternative decolonial futures.

Commentary on Case 5.2

Tineke Abma, Truus Teunissen, Doortje Kal and Gustaaf Bos

In this case the researcher is aware of her privileged position, and sensitive to the risk of reproducing existing hierarchies. She is flexible and modest in order to create space for the agendas and voices of community members, and their ways of identifying and representing themselves (as Indigenous). Co-ownership over the process of making a film and its dissemination is in line with the literature we discussed in Part 1 of this chapter. However, this is difficult to build up in a broader group of young people in a community setting, where it is difficult to have a single 'youth voice' representing all young people. How easy it would have been to take it over from them, 'speaking for' them. Not this researcher; she rather waits until they are ready, maintaining the relationships and cherishing what she has learned from them. Of course, it is a bit worrying too: doing 'good stuff' in the context of PR, but then leaving the research context after a year or two without an implementation or valorisation plan. This researcher accepts that she cannot realise change within a short period of time, and keeps hope, and expresses her solidarity with this community. This reminds us of the work of Welch (1989) who states that an 'ethic of risk' (versus an ethic of control) is not focused on results but on creating a fertile ground for protest among younger generations so that they are inspired to stay critical of oppression and marginalisation. This cannot be instructed or controlled but we can share an ethos of stamina, imagination and solidarity.

Case 5.3 Two realities meeting one another: Young service users and policy-makers in Finland

Aila-Leena Matthies

Introduction

This case comes from a university research group in Finland. It describes one action which took place in the framework of a participatory action research project: "The Role of Welfare Services for the Participatory Citizenship of the Marginalised Groups" (2011–2014), funded by the Academy of Finland. It involved a group of 20 young men, who were facing unemployment and using various welfare services. They were selected as the target group as they represent those who have been identified as the most non-participative, politically, in Finland.

The case

The project was designed so that initially the university researchers conducted focus group interviews with young people about their experiences in the services. The interviews were also a starting point for engaging them as active participants in the research. The young people then discussed the results of the focus groups and planned actions following from the results. So it was the young people who suggested, prepared and organised different actions with the support of the researchers. In the focus group interviews, young people had raised their negative experiences of using services. One of the ideas the young people suggested was to talk to those who make the decisions, as they seem not to know the consequences of their decisions for the people affected.

The discussion with the politicians and managers was organised by the university research group together with the young people, who also were the main speakers. The moderator was a practitioner from an NGO, and the young people knew her well as she worked with them in the youth café. All the members of the municipal city council and regional members of the national parliament were invited, as were regional heads of the most relevant welfare services (labour market services, youth services, social benefit office). In the end, only 10 politicians and three authorities in leading positions of services accepted the invitation. It was important that journalists were also present.

Together with the youth practitioners and the research group, the young people worked hard to realise their ideas in preparing this event. As a walkway to the meeting hall, a bureaucratic 'adventure trail' with simulation of real-life situations, including completing challenging forms or meeting unfriendly or ignorant professional practitioners, was created. The young people prepared a presentation explaining their difficult situation in the 'service jungle', the challenges they faced in accessing the labour market and their suggestions about how to improve services. Also, targeted questions to politicians were formulated, and a call was made for the decision-makers to try living for one week on the same amount of money as unemployment benefit.

For the young people this was their first chance to meet politicians and talk with them. In addition, they lacked experience in giving presentations in front of the media, which had made them extremely nervous. However, their peer group, their worker and the research group managed to encourage them and the presentation was rehearsed several times. The presentation was made by one of the leading figures of the group, and a couple of other young people added their own comments as experts by experience.

In spite of high tensions and the critical approach of the event, most of the politicians and authorities seemed to like the ideas and the presentation. They took notes carefully and asked many questions in order to learn more. It is seldom that they have the chance to listen to this kind of target group in a safe place and interactive atmosphere in regard to the decisions they make. They received useful information concerning several important topics including the national policies addressing unemployment among the young and possible solutions. The discussion was therefore mostly positive and supportive. We as researchers learned that in order to have an impact on policy-makers the authentic voice of the affected people is much more relevant than the presentations or publications of researchers.

However, one of the local politicians started to give his opinion that the young people's problems were caused by their parents, who have not taken care properly of the career development of their children: 'it's all in the home.' He also started to compare the young people with the success of his own children. Another member of the national parliament played constantly with his phone and appeared not to listen to the young people. When asked for his opinion, he suggested that going to work would be the best form of social security for these young people. We as researchers were worried about how these behaviours would hurt the young people, for whom we felt responsible. However, the moderator stopped the first politician and the second one's irrelevant comment just made all the participants laugh at him.

Some of the young people talked openly about their individual cases and were able to get the director of the services to admit that mistakes had been made. Media reports on national TV, regional radio and newspapers, including interviews with the young people, were a real success. Many positive comments were given on social media that praised the courage of the young people to speak in the name of thousands of others in the service jungle. The leading authorities also felt that they were able to get their voices heard better by the politicians, as they were supported by the voices of the young people. As a consequence of the event, the young people were invited to talk in the national parliament and one, the speaker, decided to get involved in local politics and plans to become a candidate for the municipal parliament.

The event concluded with a statement from the politicians that they had learned a lot from the young people and the authorities considered sharing the views of the young people on the prevalent issues. However, as one of the young people added: 'we may share the same opinion, but the major difference becomes reality for us when we return to our homes – you will have food in your fridge, but we will not.' As the university could not pay a direct salary to the young people for their participation, we asked them to suggest another form of compensation. They suggested a voucher for a pizzeria.

In spite of the success of the event, there were no immediate visible improvements in the young peoples' everyday lives or changes in service cultures. Instead, it became just another frustrating experience – that the politicians were all talk and no action. Although there may have been longer-term impacts, follow-up was not possible in the frame of the research.

These kinds of events linked to the PR were considered to be important settings for interaction between the worlds of the politicians and the young service users. However, striking questions remain: How ethical is it to involve people and give them hope for change if they are once again simply deceived? Did the research project actually misuse the young people for research purposes and to gain media presence for the politicians? How can research have long-term impact on the structural oppression experienced by individual unemployed people?

Commentary on Case 5.3

Tineke Abma, Truus Teunissen, Doortje Kal and Gustaaf Bos

In this case the researchers worked collaboratively with young service users to amplify their voices in the political arena. Initially, they felt a communicative space was created where they were heard. However, later on, little seemed to change right away in the lives of the people involved in line with how they had envisioned the impact. The dilemma the researchers pose is how ethical it is to create hope and expectations of change when the consequences of actions are unknown, and can be disempowering. We can see that this is frustrating when we reason from what Welch (1989) calls an 'ethic of control'. Then we are assuming that change can be controlled and results will lead to improvements in the lives of people concerned. This can then be disempowering for all involved, including the researchers. As in our reflection on Case 5.2, we think this 'ethic of control' is not very helpful here. It paralyses us, and is not realistic. It may even lead to negativity and cynicism.

We think the case demonstrates the necessity of embedding PR projects in inclusionary societal and political contexts. If before, throughout and after participatory projects there is a lack of a stimulating, welcoming and receptive context, the risk of failure is high. This is what we see happening here: the refusal of many invited people to come, the disrespectful behaviour of some attending policy-makers during the meeting, and the apparent window-dressing (words instead of actions) undermined the ability of the young service users to speak effectively for themselves.

Case 5.4 About the 'co' in co-writing: Challenges for a Dutch university researcher co-researching with people with intellectual disabilities

Gustaaf Bos and Rafaella van den Bosch

Introduction

This case is contributed by a Dutch post-doctoral university researcher (Gustaaf) and a trained researcher with an intellectual disability (Rafaella), both working on a research project that is evaluating a programme for developing experiential knowledge with people with intellectual disabilities (*mensen met een verstandelijke beperking*). The project was funded by a care institution for people with intellectual disabilities. In the Netherlands '*verstandelijke beperking*' covers a diverse range of people who need some degree of specialised care and/or support because of a (to some extent insurmountable) congenital delay in development and/or a delay in education. In everyday life people with this label often face stigmatisation, discrimination and social exclusion. The case is in two parts. It starts with the dilemmas faced by Gustaaf when writing together with Rafaella. In the second part, Rafaella reflects briefly on the issues raised by Gustaaf.

The case

Part 1: Perspectives from Gustaaf

In a participatory, responsive research design, I am conducting research together with Rafaella, a young, vibrant, intelligent woman with an intellectual disability, who is mother to three children. Rafaella receives support from a Dutch care institution for people with intellectual disabilities that funds our research project. In this project we are investigating a curriculum that aims at training 10 service users to become experts by experience. Due to this curriculum, the care organisation aims for a solid positioning of experiential expertise in everyday practice. Rafaella initially wanted to enrol in this curriculum, but when she was not selected, I seized the opportunity to ask her to become one of my co-researchers, in return for a short training and a small monthly allowance.

At the start of the project, I trained Rafaella and another person who was to become a co-researcher for five weeks in how to do responsive research, i.e. how to attend to the issues of others and how to perform participant observations and semi-structured interviews. After those five weeks, we went outside to practise and learn-by-experience. In about six months' time, we have conducted around 20 participant-observations and a dozen semi-structured interviews together.

As part of the initial training phase, Rafaella and her fellow aspirant-researcher had to write a few short assignments. In addition, after each participant-observation session I asked them to hand in a brief report. Rafaella in particular seemed very insecure about her writing abilities. Every time that she handed in a piece she had written, she would ask me to correct her 'grammatical errors and the other mistakes I made'.

But I hesitated to do so. Initially, I responded by saying I would certainly get back to her if I did not understand something, but I was not going to be her Dutch language teacher. Rafaella agreed on this, but a few weeks later she insisted that I should do a better job correcting her 'errors', because her nine-year old son had been laughing at something that she had written, in a piece I had already read. Rafaella said she felt embarrassed and she did not want to feel 'dumb', especially not in the eyes of her children.

Although I still felt unsure about this 'correcting role', I agreed to highlight grammatical errors and unusual sentence structures in her future writings, and suggest alternatives. But when I did that to one of her texts, I was struck by doubts about what I was doing. To what extent should I alter Rafaella's words? And with what justification should I correct sentence structures? Why should I correct anything that she wrote? I came to think that 'incorrect', 'authentic', 'unconventional' use of language might be symbolic for what is at stake in many interactions between people/researchers with and without intellectual disabilities. If I attached 'my' (i.e.

the culturally dominant) meaning and structure to Rafaella's writings, I would eradicate this tension, keep it out of sight. In other words, if I proceeded in this correcting role, I could be jeopardising an important condition of any writing and reading between researchers: that the reader should hold an open, attentive, curious attitude towards what is meant by the writer. From this perspective, wouldn't it (potentially) be more revealing and interesting to leave the texts unaltered?

But what might happen if I do not correct these 'flawed' texts? So far, and within the context of the care institution, we have had a lot of positive comments on the (unaltered) reports of my co-researchers. However, I am afraid about the reactions in a less understanding context, such as the academic world. Will our writing even be accepted if it contains grammatical errors?

Besides, to what extent are my co-researchers 'really' contributing to the content of a future publication, according to scientific standards? And will they be acknowledged for that – as co-authors? Related to this, there is also the issue of translating our Dutch writings into English. This translation enlarges the chance of changes in meaning, as well as a loss of control for my co-researchers – who hardly speak, write and read English. To what extent will they be able to contribute to a scientific publication that they cannot read and understand? Will they even feel free to do so?

When I discussed these issues with Rafaella, she repeated firmly that she would appreciate my correcting her 'errors', because she could learn from that. According to her, it was mainly about 'honesty' and 'shame': 'I would rather have someone, or you, being honest about my mistakes. If you leave them unaltered, and it is not written correctly, it will not be readable to others. Then I would feel ashamed – and that is the worst to me!' Rafaella said that she considered my correcting her texts as a 'promotion'. She also denied my concern about her losing control of the writing due to the English translation; 'We always have Google translate!'

Rafaella's encouraging and light-hearted response did not diminish my doubts about a correcting role. If anything, my concerns were increased: how, and with what justification, would I proceed if Rafaella and I were unable to share a definition of the issues at stake here?

Part 2: Reflections from Rafaella[1]

I really wanted that Gustaaf was honest whenever I wrote something incorrectly, and that he would adjust my spelling errors. But he thought of that as unnecessary, because he deems the way I write special. I think it is important that he corrects my errors, because I do not want people to consider my writing weird. And I would be ashamed if my children would read what I wrote and would not understand it. At the moment, I really try to do the best I can and to pay attention to how I write. That is why I thought Gustaaf should say honestly when I made writing errors.

---

1 Gustaaf translated Rafaella's response from Dutch to English, and Tineke commented on this translation and the meaning of some words. Rafaella approved the final translation.

Commentary on Case 5.4

Tineke Abma, Truus Teunissen and Doortje Kal

In this case the academic researcher wrestles with the dilemma whether or not to correct the text written by a co-researcher who feels her language does not live up to the Dutch language norm of ABN ('*Algemeen Beschaafd Nederlands*'), which translates as something like 'general highly educated Dutch'. '*Beschaafd*' stands in opposition to the primitive, not well-educated, morally underdeveloped. The researcher feels Rafaella's wish to live up to those standards leads to normalisation, and he is afraid something will get lost when her particular way of speaking and writing is corrected by him. It is clear that Rafaella feels a need to belong to what is considered 'normal'; she is ashamed of her language. The researcher negotiates with her and explains his doubts, but Rafaella persists in her wish. The researcher tries to be creative and find some middle ground, but is still searching for a working relationship that acknowledges their equity and 'humanness' as well as their difference.

There is literature on the act of translation between languages, and how this translation is always an interpretation and thus may influence the meaning of what is communicated. We should therefore be cautious, like the academic researcher in this case, in translating language (cf. Van Nes et al., 2010). There may even be some elements that are 'untranslatable' (Dahler-Larsen et al., 2016). We think this case also hints at the importance of being aware of the power of literacy and verbality, and the exclusionary impact of written language.

Regarding co-authorship of articles, the commonly accepted norm is that to be named as a co-author, someone must not only have contributed in some way to the research, but also have read, understood and had the opportunity to comment on and amend an article. It is not clear how this would work out for Rafaella in relation to an academic article in English, but thinking through the complexities and possibilities is worth the effort. Traditional norms of academic journals may not fit the complexities of PR and it is therefore important to challenge them when necessary. However, there are other options to credit the efforts of essential contributors to an article, for example in a word of thanks. It takes courage, honesty and sincerity to be clear about this to co-researchers throughout the research and writing process.

PART 3: CONCLUDING COMMENTS

Tineke Abma and Gustaaf Bos

This chapter invites readers to reflect on issues of co-ownership, dissemination and impact. Since we performed a (modest) systematic search on this topic and found few results, there appears to be some 'barren ground' left to dig deeper into these issues. It is very powerful to work with cases to further develop our moral sensitivity. Many issues discussed in the cases are everyday ethical concerns for participatory researchers, ranging from 'should I pay people who live in poor circumstances to contribute to research?' to 'should I correct the spelling of someone with an intellectual disability?' Those issues cannot be answered in general: that is, principles such as co-ownership, shared dissemination and impact give us a moral compass but always need to be interpreted in particular and concrete circumstances. As Nussbaum (2006) suggests, we have to move between general rules and particular cases. Paying attention to particulars, multiple value-commitments and perspectives, and creating spaces to reflect on these value-commitments together – thus slowing down our work – can heighten the moral goodness of our practices.

Co-ownership refers to sharing power and control over the research process, including dissemination and impact. Key issues include prevention of colonisation and co-option (promising participation but not actually and genuinely practising this). Pathways to dissemination need to be discussed early with all involved. Critical ethical issues relate to responsibility and leadership over dissemination (not necessarily the academics!), the prioritising and reaching of various audience groups (not necessarily academic peers) and issues of representation of people and their life worlds (preventing stigmatisation). Impact concerns the change PR envisions. Ethical issues relate to various, sometimes conflicting, ideas about desirable impact (preferably local change from a PR viewpoint) and non-impact on the lives and practices of those involved (partly due to the political and organisational context). Welch's (1989) 'ethic of risk' is hopeful. It acknowledges the complexity of life, and that we cannot oversee the consequences of our deeds. Furthermore, it cherishes the beauty of life and friendly, loving relationships, and sees these as an inspiration to fight for more justice. Finally, it sees the power and energy brought about by the movement of a transformation set in motion, even if it does not realise this full potential. We see such healing power in many cases. Sharing an 'ethic of risk' with co-researchers and participants is important to prevent disappointment. Obviously, this embracing of risk does not preclude participatory researchers from the moral obligation to care about the well-being of their co-researchers and research participants.

References

Abell. S., Ashmore, J., Beart, S., Brownley, P., Butcher, A., Clarke, Z., et al. (2007). Including everyone in research: The Burton Street Research Group. *British Journal of Learning Disabilities, 35*(2), 121–124.

Abma, T. A., Nierse, C. & Widdershoven, G. A. M. (2009). Patients as research partners in responsive research. Methodological notions for collaborations in research agenda setting. *Qualitative Health Research, 19*(3), 401–415.

Abma, T. A., Banks, S., Cook, T., Dias, S., Madsen, W., Springett, J., et al. (2019). *Participatory Research for Health and Social Well-Being.* Dordrecht, The Netherlands: Springer [forthcoming].

Arnstein, S. R. (1969). A ladder of citizen participation. *Journal of the American Institute of Planners, 35*(4), 216–224.

Banks, S., Armstrong, A., Carter, K., Graham, H., Hayward, P., Henry, A., et al. (2013). Everyday ethics in community-based participatory research, *Contemporary Social Science*, *8*(3), 263–277.

Banks, S., Herrington, T., & Carter, K. (2017). Pathways to co-impact: action research and community organising. *Educational Action Research*, *25*(4), 541–559.

Baur, V. E., Abma, T. A., & Widdershoven, G. A. M. (2010). Participation of marginalized groups in evaluation: mission impossible? *Evaluation and Program Planning*, *33*(3), 238–245.

Belam, J., Harris, G., Kernick, D., Kline, F., Lindley, K., McWatt J., et al. (2005). A qualitative study of migraine involving patient researchers. *The British Journal of General Practice*, *55*(511), 87–93.

Belderbos, R., Cassiman, B., Faems, D., & Leten, B.(2014). Co-ownership of intellectual property: Exploring the value-appropriation and value-creation implications of co-patenting with different partners. *Research Policy*, *43*(5), 841–852.

Benoit, C., Jansson, M., Millar, A., & Phillips, R. (2005). Community-Academic Research on Hard-to-Reach Populations: Benefits and Challenges. *Qualitative Health Research*, *15*(2), 263–282.

Beresford, P., & Russo, J. (2016). Supporting the sustainability of Mad Studies and preventing its co-option, *Disability & Society*, *31*(2), 270-274, doi: 10.1080/09687599.2016.1145380

Bos, G. F. (2016). *Antwoorden op andersheid. Over ontmoetingen tussen mensen met en zonder verstandelijke beperking in omgekeerde-integratiesettingen* [Responding to otherness: About encounters between people with and without intellectual disabilities in 'reversed integration' settings]. Nieuwegein: EPC.

Bos, G. F. & Kal, D. (2016). The value of inequality. *Social Inclusion*, *4*(4), 129–139.

Boumans, J. (2012). Het subject als maatstaf? Een essay over de valkuilen van het onderzoek naar ervaringskennis. [The subject as measuring stick? An essay on the pitfalls of research into experiential knowledge.] In J. Jansen, (red.), T. Dobbelaar (red.), *Zie meer, kijk anders. Tien jonge wetenschappers over disability studies* (pp. 71–85). [See more, look differently: Ten young scientists on disability studies.] The Hague: ZonMw.

Brabeck, K., Lykes, M. B., Sibley, E., & Kene, P. (2015). Ethical ambiguities in participatory action research with unauthorized migrants. *Ethics & Behavior*, *25*, 21–36.

Bromley, E., Mikesell, L., Jones, F., & Khodyakov, D. (2015). From subject to participant: Ethics and the evolving role of community in health research. *American Journal of Public Health*, *105*, 900–908.

Brugge, D., & Cole, A. (2003). A case study of community-based participatory research ethics: The healthy public housing initiative. *Science & Engineering Ethics*, *9*, 485–501.

Buckley, B., Grant, A. M., Firkins, L., Greene A. C., & Frankau, J. (2007). Working together to identify research questions. *Continence UK*, *1*(1), 76–81.

Burkitt, I. (2015). Relational agency. Relational sociology, agency and interaction. *European Journal of Social Theory*, *19*(3), 322–339.

Byrne, E., Elliot, E., & Williams, G. (2015). Poor places, powerful people? Co-producing cultural counter-representations of place. *Visual Methodologies*, *3*(2), 77–85.

Caron-Flinterman, J. F., Broerse, J. E. W., Teerling, J., & Bunders, J. F. G. (2005). Patients' priorities concerning health research: the case of asthma and COPD research in the Netherlands. *Health Expectations*, *8*(3), 253–263.

Cook, T. (2009). The purpose of mess in action research: Building rigour through a messy turn. *Educational Action Research*, *17*(2), 277–291.

Cook, T. & Roche, B. (Eds.) (2017). The conceptualisation and articulation of impact:

hopes, expectations and challenges for the participatory paradigm [Special Issue]. *Educational Action Research*, 25(4).

Coulter, A. & Ellins, J. (2007). Effectiveness of strategies for informing, educating and involving patients. *British Medical Journal*, *335*(7609), 24–27.

Dahler-Larsen, P., Abma, T. A., Bustelo, M., Irimia, R., Kosunen, S., et al. (2016). Evaluation, language and untranslatables, *American Journal of Evaluation*, *38*(1), 1–12.

Durham Community Research Team. (2011). *Community-based Participatory Research: Ethical Challenges*. Durham: Centre for Social Justice and Community Action, Durham University, www.dur.ac.uk socialjustice/researchprojects/cbpr/ (accessed January 2018).

Eccles, M. P., Grimshaw, J. M., Shekelle, P., Schünemann, H. J., & Woolf, F. (2012). Developing clinical practice guidelines: target audiences, identifying topics for guidelines, guideline group composition and functioning and conflicts of interest. *Implementation Science*, 7: 60.

Entwistle, V. A., Renfrew, M. J., Yearley, S., Forrester, J., & Lamont, T. (1998). Lay perspectives: advantages for health research. *British Medical Journal*, *316*(7129), 463–466.

Faulkner A., & Thomas, P. (2002). User-led research and evidence-based medicine. *British Journal of Psychiatry*, *180*, 1–3.

Fricker, M. (2007). *Epistemic Injustice: Power and the Ethics of Knowing*. Oxford: Oxford University Press.

Gilchrist, A. (2015). *Community voices research – AHRC co-design projects: Implications for academics and funders*. Cardiff: Cardiff University, AHRC Connected Communities research programme.

Gilligan, C. (1982). *In a Different Voice*. Cambridge, Mass: Harvard University Press.

Greene, S. (2013). Peer research assistantships and the ethics of reciprocity in community-based research. *Journal of Empirical Research on Human Research Ethics*, *8*, 141–152.

Groot, B. C., Haveman, A., Huberts, M., Schout, G. Vink, M. & Abma, T. A. (2018) Ethics of care in participatory health research. Mutual responsibility in collaboration with co-researchers, *Educational Action Research*, published online, https://doi.org/10.1080/0 9650792.2018.1450771

Guba, E.G. & Lincoln, Y.S. (1989). *Fourth generation evaluation*. Beverly Hills: Sage.

Hellstrom, I., Nolan, M., Nordenfelt, L., & Lundh, U. (2007). Ethical and Methodological Issues in Interviewing Persons With Dementia. *Nursing Ethics*, *14*(5), 608–619.

Kal, D. (2001). Kwartiermaken. Werken aan ruimte voor mensen met een psychiatrische achtergrond ['Setting up camp': Preparing a welcome for people with a psychiatric background]. Amsterdam: Boom.

Kal, D. (2012). Kwartiermaken, creating space for otherness. In H. van Ewijk, J. van Eijken, & H. Staatsen (Eds.), *A good society is more than just a private affair. Citizenship based social work in practice. Studies in comparative social pedagogies and international social work and social policy* (pp. 25–41). Bremen: EHV.

Knox, M., Mok, M., & Parmenter, T.R. (2000). Working with the experts: collaborative research with people with an intellectual disability. *Disability & Society*, *15*(1), 49–61.

Marsden J., & Bradburn, J. (2004). Patient and clinician collaboration in the design of a national randomized breast cancer trial. *Health Expectations*, *7*(1), 6–17.

Mitchell, T. L., & Baker, E. (2005). Community-building versus career-building research: The challenges, risks, and responsibilities of conducting research with Aboriginal and Native American communities. *Journal of Cancer Education*, *20*, 41–46.

McVilly, K. R., Stancliffe, R. J., Parmenter, T. R., & Burton-Smith, R. M. (2006). Self-advocates have the last say on friendship. *Disability & Society*, *21*(7), 693–708.

Nierse, C. & Abma, T. A. (2011). Developing voice and empowerment: the first step towards a broad consultation in research agenda setting. *Journal of Intellectual Disability Research*, *55*(4), 411–21.

Nussbaum, M. C. (2006). *Frontiers of Justice: Disability, Nationality, Species Membership*. Cambridge, MA: Harvard University Press, Belknap Press.

Pain, R., Askins, K., Banks, S., Cook, T., Crawford, G., et al. (2015). *Mapping Alternative Impact: Alternative approaches to impact from co-produced research*, www.dur.ac.uk/socialjus tice/researchprojects/mapping-alt-impact/ (accessed 14 November 2017)

Quigley, D. (2006). A review of improved ethical practices in environmental and public health research: Case examples from native communities. *Health Education and Behavior*, *33*(2), 130–147.

Richardson M. (2000). How we live: participatory research with six people with learning difficulties. *Journal of Advanced Nursing*, *32*(6), 1383–1395.

Rink, E., Montgomery-Andersen, R., Koch, A., Mulvad, G., & Gesink, D. (2013). Ethical challenges and lessons learned from Inuulluataarneq – 'Having the good life' study: A community-based participatory research project in Greenland. *Journal of Empirical Research on Human Research Ethics*, *8*, 110–118.

Rose, D. (2017). Service user/survivor-led research in mental health: epistemological possibilities, *Disability & Society*, *32*(6), 773–789.

Russo, J. & Beresford, P. (2015). Between exclusion and colonisation: seeking a place for mad people's knowledge in academia. *Disability & Society*, *30*(1), 153–157.

Schipper, K., Bakker, M., De Wit, M., Ket, J.C.F., & Abma, T.A. (2016). Strategies for dis- seminating recommendations or guidelines to patients: a systematic review, *Implementation Science*, *11*, 82.

Schneider, B., Scissons, H., Arney, L., Benson, G., Derry, J., Lucas, K., et al. (2004). Communication Between People With Schizophrenia and Their Medical Professionals: A Participatory Research Project. *Qualitative Health Research*, *14*(4), 562–577.

Staniszewska, S., Jones, N., Newburn, M., & Marshall, S. (2007). User involvement in the development of a research bid: barriers, enablers and impacts. *Health Expectations*, *10*(2), 173–183.

Teti, M., Murray, C., Johnson, L., & Binson, D. (2012). Photovoice as a community-based participatory research method among women living with HIV/AIDS: Ethical opportu- nities and challenges. *Journal of Empirical Research on Human Research Ethics*, *7*(4), 34–43.

Teunissen, G. J., Visse, M.A., & Abma, T. A. (2013). Struggling between strength and vul- nerability: A patient's counter story. *Health Care Analysis*, *23*(3): 288–305.

Turner, K., & Gillard, S. (2012). 'Still out there?' Is the service user voice becoming lost as user involvement moves into the mental health research mainstream? In: M. Barnes and P. Cotterell (Eds). *Critical perspectives on user involvement*, (pp. 189–201). Bristol: The Policy Press.

Van Nes, F., Abma, T. A., Jonsson, H., & Deeg, D. (2010) Language differences in qual- itative research. Is meaning lost in translation? *European Journal of Aging Studies*, *7*(4), 313–316.

Vishalache, B., & Cornforth, S. (2013). Using working agreements in participatory action research: Working through moral problems with Malaysian students. *Educational Action Research*, *21*, 582–602.

Waldenfels, B. (2004). Bodily experience between selfhood and otherness. *Phenomenology and the Cognitive Sciences*, *3*, 235–248.

Walsh, C. A., Hewson, J., Shier, M., & Morales, E. (2008). Unraveling ethics: Reflections from a community-based participatory research project with youth. *Qualitative Report*, *13*, 379–393.

Welch, S. D. (1989). *A feminist ethic of risk*. Minneapolis: Augsburg Fortress Publishing.

White, M.A. & Verhoef, M.J. (2005). Toward a Patient-Centered Approach: Incorporating Principles of Participatory Action Research into Clinical Studies. *Integrative Cancer Therapies*, 4(1), 21–24.

Williams, R. L., Willging, C. E., Quintero, G., Kalishman, S., Sussman, A. L. et al. (2010). Ethics of Health Research in Communities: Perspectives From the Southwestern United States. *Annals of Family Medicine*, 8(5), 433–439.

Wilson, E., Kenny, A., & Dickson-Swift, V. (2018). Ethical Challenges in Community-Based Participatory Research: A Scoping Review. *Qualitative Health Research*, 28(2), 189–199.

6

ANONYMITY, PRIVACY, AND CONFIDENTIALITY

Kristin Kalsem

With cases contributed by Alana Martin, Christine Lalonde, Lisa Boucher, Claire Kendall, Zack Marshall, Sarah Switzer, Carol Strike, Adrian Guta, Soo Chan Carusone, Michele Brear, and Vu Song Ha.

PART 1: INTRODUCTION AND OVERVIEW OF ISSUES

Background

Trust between researchers and participants is paramount in any research project. A primary element of that trust is that agreed-upon measures relating to anonymity, privacy, and confidentiality be respected and maintained. This chapter will discuss anonymity, privacy, and confidentiality in the specific context of participatory research (PR), examining why traditional ethical models for thinking about these aspects of human subjects research do not "fit" easily with PR, as well as the particular challenges that participatory researchers face in determining the extent to which anonymity, privacy, and confidentiality are desirable and even possible in light of the very nature of PR.

The first part of this chapter will discuss the concepts of anonymity, privacy, and confidentiality more generally in the context of human subjects research. It will then highlight why and how the ideological premises of PR as well as its methodologies can be in tension with more traditional approaches to addressing anonymity, privacy, and confidentiality in research. Suggestions of ways that may be helpful to think about or address these issues also will be presented. The second part of this chapter includes four case studies that raise various ethical issues on these topics. Case 6.1 discusses how a research team in Ottawa, Canada handled issues of anonymity, privacy, and confidentiality when research equipment was stolen and data was compromised. The stolen equipment included five taped interviews, each of which included identifying and private information. Case 6.2 relates to a community-based research project at a small sub-acute HIV hospital in Toronto, Canada. In this study, the small size of the community, the hospital setting, and the complicated line between clinical care and research presented challenges to anonymity, privacy, and confidentiality. In Case 6.3, a researcher working with community co-researchers in a rural village in Swaziland discusses the ethical dilemma of not being able to recognise the work of the co-researchers without compromising the anonymity, privacy, and confidentiality of other participants and the community. The case study reveals the need for ongoing and nuanced discussions about the context of disclosing the co-researchers, other participants, and the community to find the most appropriate balance between more traditional ethical obligations and the ethical obligation in PR of equitably recognising the team's contributions. Case 6.4 explores issues of anonymity, privacy, and confidentiality that arose in a PhotoVoice project conducted in Hanoi, Vietnam with teenagers with Autism Spectrum Disorder (ASD). It discusses the views and perspectives of the children and their parents on the value and risks of using the teenagers' real names and identifying information at a public exhibit planned to raise awareness of ASD, as well as in academic publications.

I will offer a short commentary after each case study, analysing the specific concerns raised in that particular situation within the larger ethical conversation of anonymity, privacy, and confidentiality in PR. As a legal scholar, I can be very focused on privacy-related concerns and obligations, as well as the specific terms of an informed consent. However, as a legal researcher who engages primarily in community-based problem solving using PR methods, I am well aware of the complicating factors that arise when rules established for a certain type of more traditional study cannot easily be adapted to different sets of circumstances.

The concepts: anonymity, privacy, and confidentiality

While distinct from one another, the concepts of anonymity, privacy, and confidentiality are often discussed together and blurred. There is no one or precise definition for any of the terms; their meanings are context dependent. As a starting point for considering the ethical issues that arise relating to anonymity, privacy, and confidentiality, this chapter will set out some general ways that researchers think about each of these concepts when conducting research on human subjects.

Anonymity, in the research context, generally means that the identity of the participant will be protected. In an anonymous study, there should be no way to associate a particular person with particular data or to even know that a particular person has participated in the study at all (Pritchard, 2002). Common practises to ensure anonymity involve assigning pseudonyms, aggregating identifiers, describing the characteristics of participants in ranges (e.g., ages 18–25), and using anonymised quotations (Morse, 1998; Wiles, Charles, Crow, & Heath, 2006).

Library shelves are filled with books and treatises devoted to the meanings of *privacy*. As a legal scholar, I often am dealing with 'the right to privacy', and thinking about ways in which people's lives should not be interfered with by the government or other individuals. For purposes of considering ethical issues relating to privacy and research, however, I think it is more relevant to speak of what

W.A. Parent describes as 'the condition of privacy' and defines as 'not having undocumented personal knowledge about one possessed by others' (1983, p. 269). Since this definition of 'undocumented' means not available in any public record, it provides a helpful way to consider what it means for a researcher to discover personal knowledge that is not yet (and that the participant might not ever want to be) made part of a public record (such as a research publication). What might a person want to keep private? Parent describes such personal knowledge as consisting of

> facts which most persons in a given society choose not to reveal about themselves (except to close friends, family, . . .) or of facts about which a particular individual is acutely sensitive and which he therefore does not choose to reveal about himself, even though most people don't care if these same facts are widely known about themselves.
>
> *(1983, p. 270)*

It is important to keep in mind that research participants may have a wide spectrum of privacy concerns.

In research, the focus of anonymity is the participant, whereas the focus of *confidentiality* usually is the data (Wiles et al., 2006). In many studies, the researchers know who the participants are and who has provided what information. They may, however, agree to keep that information confidential, to protect what is shared from disclosure (Pritchard, 2002). Moreover, Easter, Davis, and Henderson (2004) offer a helpful distinction between confidentiality and privacy: 'Although often conflated under the rubric of "confidentiality," setting privacy and confidentiality out separately makes clear that they are important and discrete concepts: privacy, freedom from having private facts made public, and confidentiality, keeping shared information within a relationship' (13–14). In other words, there is trust that, even though researchers may learn private information from or about a participant whom they can identify, they will use that data only according to agreed-upon terms of confidentiality. This commitment to confidentiality has both 'instrumental' and 'intrinsic' value:

> As an instrumental value, the purpose is to protect subjects from the specific harms that might come from disclosure, e.g., loss of insurance or employment, or embarrassment. By contrast, confidentiality as an intrinsic value is a commitment to respect persons.
>
> *(Easter et al., 2004, p. 13)*

In some research, it may be possible to keep data confidential but not maintain anonymity. Privacy may be more important to some participants than others. The agreed-upon terms between the researchers and participants relating to anonymity, privacy, and confidentiality usually are set out in an informed consent form, signed by the participants at the beginning of the research project. Rather than relying on a boilerplate paragraph relating to these concepts, it is prudent for researchers to tailor the language as best they can to fit the specific circumstances of the research.

As will be discussed later in this chapter, PR requires that ongoing attention be paid to these issues as the specific directions and methods of the research may change over time.

Because of the ways in which PR differs from more traditional studies involving human subjects, it is necessary to think differently about what the categories of anonymity, privacy, and confidentiality mean, how participants can be appropriately protected and respected, and how trust can be established and maintained throughout the course of the research. Ideologically, for example, PR is committed to stakeholder participation. What does anonymity mean in that context? Is it even possible? PR has proven very effective in gathering data from "at risk" or "hard to reach" communities such as the HIV patients discussed in Case 6.2 and the community members in rural Africa discussed in Case 6.3. How does that complicate privacy concerns? PR often is conducted in the first place to effect real change in a local community. How might the actions that grow out of the research impact agreed-upon terms of confidentiality? The next section explores some of the complexities of these PR-related ethical issues.

Ethical issues relating to anonymity, privacy, and confidentiality

In this chapter, the following four aspects of PR that present particularly complex ethical issues regarding anonymity, privacy, and confidentiality will be examined:

- In PR, there often is no clear-cut separation between researcher and researched.
- The design of PR means the scope and direction(s) of the research are not determined and set at the outset.
- PR is very concerned about power relationships, including what is done with the data and who is given credit for the research.
- PR involves activism and social change.

With respect to each of these salient features of PR, this chapter will highlight how and why difficult ethical challenges arise, as well as present suggestions of best practises that may be helpful in certain research scenarios.

In PR, there often is no clear-cut separation between researcher and researched.

Thus far in this chapter, I have made a distinction between 'researcher' and 'participant'. In introducing more general understandings of anonymity, privacy, and confidentiality, this distinction, which is typical in most human subjects research, made sense. This clear distinction, however, is not typical at all in PR.

A real strength of PR is that participants often are co-researchers. They are likely to be involved at all stages, from helping to identify the research questions in the first place to determining methodologies, to gathering and disseminating data, to ultimately implementing change based on the research findings. Immediately one can see how this challenges traditional rules or codes of ethics. Just thinking about anonymity in this situation can be mindboggling. Who is to be anonymous to whom for example? Who can remain anonymous and who cannot and what does that mean? Van den Hoonaard goes so far as to say that anonymity in ethnographic and qualitative research is 'a virtual impossibility' (2003, p. 141).

In an article entitled 'Research Ethics Committees and Participatory Action Research with Young People: The Politics of Voice', a group of young women from East London (UK) discussed their frustrations with strict requirements often imposed by ethics committees that the identities of persons under 18 be kept anonymous. They were co-researchers in a PR study investigating young people's sense of political agency. These young women wanted recognition for their work and it was important to them to voice their own thoughts and interpretations of the research findings. Appreciating the beneficial ways that PR has of empowering marginalised groups like young people, the women noted that 'given the even greater power imbalance between young "subjects" and adult researchers, when compared with adult "subjects" and researchers, it is arguably especially progressive to enable youthful participation in research processes' (Yanar et al., 2016, p. 123). This made it all the more problematic that 'the well-meaning paternalism underpinning the requirement for anonymity is fundamentally at odds with the enabling ethics underpinning PAR methodologies' (Yanar et al., 2016, p. 124).

Of course, the very fact that the young women were able to write and be named in the published article illustrates that it may be possible and well worth the while to approach the governing ethics board with a well-argued position of why a particular rule is not only unnecessary in a specific PR study, but may actually have detrimental effects. Brydon-Miller and Greenwood (2006), for example, have found that ethics review boards may be open to rethinking certain requirements as they become more familiar with PR (see also Chapter 7 this volume).

There are tricky issues not only of anonymity but also privacy and confidentiality when the research team comprises members of the community that is being researched. Community-based researchers often can be the best collectors of data precisely because they are members of a given community. They have the trust of the community that is the 'subject' of the research because they are part of it. But if these community members are gathering data as co-researchers, their own identities are not anonymous – people know they are contributing to the research. Moreover, as Merritt et al. highlight,

> The very event of a home visit by a field worker has the potential to breach a subject's confidentiality by exposing private circumstances to the neighborhood, as when a field worker tests a subject for pregnancy and brings antenatal supplements on subsequent visits.
>
> *(2010, p. 2)*

Merritt et al. also highlight, however, that the very fact that PR trains community members in research ethics, including the importance of informed consent, has the potential benefit of making issues of anonymity, privacy, and confidentiality (including risks associated with participating in the research) more open to discussion and consent more truly informed.

The difficult ethical dilemmas relating to anonymity, privacy, and confidentiality can be integrated into the research training for the PR project itself, creating a heightened awareness of tensions upfront. The initial training also presents an opportunity to think through as a team what potential issues on these topics are likely to arise, as well as to consider what to do when unanticipated circumstances develop.

The design of PR means the scope and direction(s) of the research are not determined and set at the outset.

PR is designed to allow for the research to proceed organically. At the beginning of a project, the research question itself may not be certain, let alone what the methods and next steps might be. Whether and how anonymity, privacy, and confidentiality will be possible, and on what terms, is often up in the air at the time a participant is asked to give informed consent. Compounding this is the fact that more traditional methods of protecting identities and data do not work (or need to be adapted) when using several methodologies frequently used in PR.

While it is one thing to speak of anonymity, for example, when the participants are filling out a survey, it is quite another when they are gathered together and individuals share personal information as part of a group interaction. Relatedly, while steps can be taken to keep information shared in group settings (data) confidential from others who are not present, it is not confidential with respect to the others present at the time. Even if information is not shared in a group setting, if, as is often the case with PR, the 'community' being studied is relatively small, it is possible that certain details shared will make an individual identifiable to others in a small-knit community.

Moreover, as Pritchard explains, qualitative methods generally may uncover unexpected private information:

> Practitioner researchers spend considerable time with their subjects, asking questions and observing events in the natural flow of activity, rather than adhering to a set operational plan. Things are said, events happen, and information comes to light that were not anticipated.
>
> *(2002, p. 4)*

What to do when such information is discovered can create complex ethical issues regarding privacy and confidentiality, as well as legal issues, for example, when there is mandatory reporting of child abuse.

Even if a researcher does not know and therefore is unable to inform the participants about all aspects of the research project at the outset, letting them know what he or she *does* know at the time likely will make it easier to work with participants if additional issues of anonymity, privacy, or confidentiality arise in the future. A detailed explanation of how PR works also will help participants understand why circumstances might change. A participant who understands the nature of the process and the reasoning behind it may feel more of a buy-in to the research and outcomes. In this way, addressing the 'problems' created by the openness and flexibility of PR may, in fact, provide opportunities to more fully engage and empower participants.

PR is very concerned about power relationships, including what is done with the data and who is given credit for the research.

PR consciously works to dismantle the typical power relationships that exist between those conducting a study and those being studied. There is an ideological commitment to the understanding that everyone has unique contributions to make and are 'experts' in different areas. Academic researchers bring certain skills and experiences to a project, but so do community members whose everyday lives are affected by the topic of the research. Ongoing attention needs to be paid to power dynamics as the study develops: 'In participatory research, the researcher must not just be cautious about the use of power, but must actively work to redistribute power and create both dialogue and equality in decision making' (Stuart, 1998, p. 305).

This sharing of power means that participant co-researchers should have a voice in how to address some of the complex ethical issues regarding anonymity, privacy, and confidentiality that arise during the research. This may be especially difficult when academic researchers have requirements from their institutional review boards or ethics committees that the community co-researchers may not think promote the best outcome. For example, in Case 6.3, community members of the African village were concerned that maintaining the anonymity of their community would mean that the results of the study could not be used to apply for funding to address the very issues that the study had brought to light. PR's training in the actual research process, including what ethical rules may need to be followed and why, may help to identify conflicts early and possibly facilitate steps that could be taken to ameliorate these issues. As discussed later in connection with the PhotoVoice exhibit presented in Case 6.4, it also may be helpful to include the community co-researchers in discussions with governing ethics bodies.

And what if, as in the previously discussed East London study (Yanar et al., 2016), participant co-researchers want credit for their research? In that case, the young women wanted to publish their research using their own names. While their circumstances were complicated by anonymity rules relating to their ages, other issues of anonymity, privacy, and confidentiality also can arise when participants want their work publicly acknowledged. For example, would acknowledging some of the participants inadvertently disclose the participation of or other private information about others? As Cases 6.3 and 6.4 below illustrate, ethical rules that are designed to protect may, instead, be disempowering, working directly in opposition to a guiding principle of PR. As Bradley explains:

> By controlling the models of research, who gets to speak and how subjects get to represent themselves, IRBs [Institutional Review Boards] are in a powerful position as part of the institutional structure. In this position they can, and often do, silence the voices of the marginalised and perpetuate an academic political economy and a traditional top-down research and professional model that quantify and objectify human lives by keeping them nameless, faceless, and voiceless.
>
> *(2007, p. 341)*

PR is about dismantling these power relationships, which may result in complex ethical dilemmas when other concerns need to be weighed against the value of empowering individuals and communities.

PR involves activism and social change.

A goal of PR is bringing about positive change. Often, PR is a method used to address community problems, with those in the community being actively involved in all stages of the research and in implementing solutions. The results are real-world, affecting the everyday lives of those in the community.

Because the community itself may be the place that the findings are reported and put into practical use, depending on the size of the community, participants may be able to be recognised and identified. Sometimes this may have deleterious effects on participants, particularly if solutions threaten those who have power and want to maintain the status quo (Lincoln & Guba, 1989; Pritchard, 2002). Social change involves *change* and not everyone may be on board.

The 'action' component of PR also may be in tension with traditional research practises regarding anonymity, privacy, and confidentiality. For example, how is it possible to facilitate marginalised people's voices and empower them politically without anyone knowing who they are? These concerns and tensions need to be part of early community conversations on what actions should be considered. If the implications that each action has with respect to anonymity, privacy, and confidentiality are taken into account, certain action agendas might make more sense than others. Would an insistence on anonymity, for example, hinder the political impact? Are there ways upfront to structure the research to balance protections with activism? In Case 6.4, privacy and anonymity concerns complicated the ways in which the action phase of educating the public on Autism Spectrum Disorder through a PhotoVoice project could be implemented. The researcher and the participants, however, were able to work together as a team to put on a successful PhotoVoice exhibit while honouring differing levels of comfort with disclosure of personal information. As community members may be in the best position to understand the risks and benefits of not insisting on strict or inflexible rules regarding anonymity, privacy, and confidentiality, they need to be informed and consulted. Being part of the process in this way also is respectful and empowering and builds trust.

In the next part of this chapter, four real-world examples of ethical issues that have arisen while doing PR and the reflections of some of the researchers involved are presented. After each case study, I will offer a brief commentary, tying some of these specific examples to the broader issues raised concerning anonymity, privacy, and confidentiality in PR.

PART 2: CASES AND COMMENTARIES

Case 6.1 Handling a privacy breach and participant notification: Challenges for a community-based research project with people who use drugs in Ottawa, Canada

Alana Martin, Christine Lalonde, Lisa Boucher, Claire Kendall, and Zack Marshall

Introduction

This case is written by a Peer Research Coordinator, a Peer Research Associate, a Research Assistant, and two Principal Investigators involved in a community-based participatory research project focusing on harm reduction among people who use drugs (PWUD) in Ottawa, Canada. The city in which this study took place has high rates of HIV and hepatitis C among PWUD. In addition to substance use experience, this community tends to experience comorbid mental health diagnoses or physical illness, poverty, unstable housing, criminalisation, and discrimination/ stigmatisation. This case is written from the perspective of the Peer Research Coordinator and one of the Peer Research Associates involved in the study. Peer Research Associates, in this case people with lived experience of substance use and marginalisation, have been actively involved in all phases of the project including study design and development of data collection tools, recruitment, survey administration and interviewing, data analysis, knowledge exchange, and overall coordination of the initiative. They were recruited from the study Community Advisory Committee and through partnerships with community organisations and by word-of-mouth. All Peer Research Associates received extensive research training including hands-on practice, as well as peer support from the Peer Research Coordinator throughout the project, and were paid for their work.

The case

The present case example outlines the difficulties experienced in navigating a privacy breach, and in particular the importance of having people with lived experience involved in notifying the affected participants.

Early in the data collection phase, we experienced a theft of petty cash funds and study equipment, including an audio recorder containing sensitive information from five participant interviews. The interviews mainly detailed participants' use of drugs and health or social services, places lived, criminal activities, important people in their lives, and aspects of their mental and physical health. A few recordings included full names and the hepatitis C status of participants. Police investigated the scene, and the Principal Investigators and core staff (including the Peer Research Coordinator) held a meeting to discuss options and decide how to proceed.

Initially we were shocked to learn about the privacy breach, and uncertain about the impact it would have for continuing the study as well as for research among our local community of PWUD more broadly. We wondered whether this incident could jeopardise the viability of the project, such as through the loss of Research Ethics Board (REB) approval, or whether it could affect our ability to receive funding for future projects. We also worried there might be an impact on our established partnerships with many community organisations, and were concerned the incident could exacerbate the hesitance already present among many people in the wider community with respect to working with PWUD. Additionally, it was hard not to feel a sense of personal guilt, as if we and our team members who are representing the community of PWUD were somehow at fault.

On the recommendation of the institutional REB, the privacy breach halted all project activities for approximately one month. During this period, the Principal Investigators and staff worked with the REB and privacy officials to ensure all necessary actions were completed. This led to much uncertainty and disturbance in the lives of our Peer Research Associate team members, including loss of income. Although the team members had grown very supportive of one another through their involvement in the study, the incident caused a temporary disruption to these working relationships. As such, we took on the responsibility of mediating inter-actions among team members to reduce the potential for unnecessary accusations.

The central issue stemming from the privacy breach involved determining how to navigate notifying the affected participants. Although these participants are part of a population that is difficult to reach for follow-up, we were able to use our established local connections to find and engage the affected participants fairly easily. The study team believed it was essential for its peer members to approach these participants, partly because our team is highly focused on developing capacity for people with lived experience to be involved in all research activities. In addi-tion, we, as Peer Research Coordinator and Peer Research Associate, were the individuals chosen to complete this task because the team considers us to be well respected in the local community, as well as able to communicate clearly while responding to participants' needs in a tactful manner.

One of the main concerns included how we would ensure that participants understood the facts and potential consequences surrounding the privacy breach. Our team prepared a two-page privacy breach notification sheet which we shared with each participant. When meeting in person, we had to determine how to translate each important point from this sheet into accessible language, as we could not be certain of literacy levels. To accomplish this, we verbally explained each point in our own words and engaged the participants in discussion to gain a sense of their understanding.

Our other main concern was how the participants and the local community would respond to this information. We were initially nervous about the potential for interpersonal conflict or negative responses on the part of participants whose interview recordings had been taken. Part of our concerns was linked to histories of criminalisation and chronic stigmatisation. Because the police were involved in investigating the incident, we made sure participants knew that their identities would not be revealed. In addition, we wondered if the privacy breach might deter PWUD from participating in similar studies due to viewing researchers as less trustworthy or not careful with their personal data.

We took an individualised approach to notifying the participants to ensure that each was aware of the specific pieces of sensitive information they had shared. As we had saved copies of the interviews, we were able to listen to them in preparation for notifying each participant.

We were fortunate that the participants' reactions were highly supportive. Overall, they were not upset about the possible personal consequences of the privacy breach. Instead, they mainly expressed concern about how the incident might impact the study, and how it could affect similar community-based participatory research (CBPR) studies in the local area. In addition, they were concerned for our personal situations, such as whether it might negatively affect our peer research jobs, as well as for the future involvement of peer workers in the community in any context (e.g., within both research and service provision).

Some researchers worry about possible risks of conducting CBPR, such as those experienced by our study team. Our case highlights the resilience of Peer Research Associates, the trust their role brings to CBPR studies, and the commitment and support of communities when they feel engaged in the research process. We hope our case can provide an example for other CBPR groups facing similar circumstances in the future.

Commentary on Case 6.1

Kristin Kalsem

This case involves issues of not only privacy, but also confidentiality and anonymity. There are privacy concerns because personal information that was not publicly available fell into the hands of the people who stole the equipment and, thus, potentially could be disclosed. Much of this information was of a sensitive nature—drug use, criminal activities, hepatitis C status—that the participants likely did not want revealed. Since the data was no longer under the exclusive control of the research team, confidentiality of the information collected also was at risk. Finally, because some of the interviewees were identified by their full names, as well as the fact that the interviews themselves may have included details specific enough to identify the interviewees, anonymity also was compromised.

Of course, no researchers plan on having their data stolen. While all steps should be taken to protect against this contingency, situations may arise like this one where the totally unexpected does indeed happen. The researchers here acted quickly, immediately notifying the research ethics board and complying with its instruction to temporarily halt the project. They report that they worked with the ethics board and privacy officials to ensure other regulatory compliance. I imagine this also included reviewing the terms of the consent forms signed by the participants to see what obligations were owing to them in the case of compromised anonymity, privacy, and confidentiality. In this case, however, it does not seem that the research ethics board took decision making away from the research team. Instead, the team worked together, making the most of the community participation that so defines PR, to make the best of an unfortunate situation.

In this case, one of the real strengths of PR is highlighted in that it was much easier to actually locate the participants whose privacy had been breached. The peer researchers had more access to them than, for example, a research team not embedded in the community might have had. Also, much thought was put in to the best way to notify the participants and to make sure that they fully understood what had happened and what risks that posed. The team's decision to have the peer researchers talk to the participants reflects the understanding that they likely have greater insight into how the participants might feel in this situation and what would show the most respect as well as help to rebuild trust. Individual care was taken to review the back-up copies of the interviews so that each participant knew what personal information about them was potentially disclosed. Also, the two-page fact sheet was not just handed out but explained with the specific purpose of making certain that the particular individual understood the information it contained.

In taking full responsibility for the breach, explaining in detail the circumstances and consequences, the research team made the participants feel informed and respected. The fact that the participants were so concerned about the impact of the theft on the study itself speaks to the success of the researchers in engaging and investing them in the work. To the participants, the risks to them of the breach were outweighed by what they felt was the value of the study. They knew that their participation mattered.

While this research team successfully navigated a potentially devastating event, this case study brings home the fact that, as researchers, we need to be aware and ask ourselves the difficult question – what if our research does find its way into unauthorised hands? Are there small changes we could make to minimise the potential harm of that? After reading about this situation, for example, I know I will be more thoughtful in the future about whether it is necessary for individuals to identify themselves by name in a taped interview. Specific identifying information might best be recorded elsewhere. It seems wise to not only consider how to avoid possible thefts or leaks of information, but also to ask the difficult 'what if' questions in the planning stages.

Case 6.2 Issues of confidentiality in working between research and clinical care: Community-based research in an HIV hospital in Toronto, Canada

Sarah Switzer, Carol Strike, Adrian Guta, Soo Chan Carusone

Introduction

This case explores issues of confidentiality, managing roles between researchers and clinicians and avoiding harm within the context of a community-based research (CBR) project at an HIV hospital in Toronto, Canada. It is written from the perspective of the research project coordinator, Sarah Switzer, who is now a PhD candidate, but with input from the study investigators.

The case

In 2010, a team of researchers at the Dalla Lana School of Public Health, University of Toronto, were approached by Casey House, a 13-bed sub-acute HIV hospital in Toronto that serves clients facing a range of complex health conditions, to collaborate with the clinical management team in order to develop a CBR study. The study was funded by a CBR and evaluation fund, which aimed to enhance the capacity of community-based HIV/AIDS organisations, their staff, and people living with HIV/AIDS, to participate meaningfully in CBR or evaluation.

The objectives of the study were to explore the hospital's newly introduced harm reduction policy and assess the feasibility of using CBR in a hospital setting. Prior to designing the study, the researchers consulted with clients on the relevance and design of the project. Clients communicated that the study aims were important, and that they were particularly interested in using arts-based approaches to engage in research questions. However, clients advised the team that while they were interested in the study, their health conditions prohibited them from extensive participation.

The research team included two academic researchers from Dalla Lana School of Public Health, a director of research (with academic training, but employed by the hospital), and a clinical manager. Other clinicians (social workers and a recreation therapist) advised on the project where needed. Members of the hospital community were living with advanced HIV and other health issues, including substance use, cognitive challenges, and other comorbidities, making it difficult for them to remember appointments without assistance and support. I (Sarah) had recently been hired as a research coordinator and was supervised by both principal investigators of the project (who occupied research and clinical positions). The research coordination office was on-site in the hospital so that we could build relationships with the community (clinicians and clients), more easily consult with clients, arrange advisory meetings, and conduct recruitment and data collection.

Based on feedback from clients, an informal and flexible community advisory board comprised of current and former clients was constructed to consult on research design, recruitment, and findings. These meetings were co-facilitated by the research coordinator and select members of the research team; they did not include clinicians involved in the project. The clients identified photography as a primary art medium for the project, leading the research team to develop a modified version of PhotoVoice. In PhotoVoice, participants are given cameras to identify, document, and analyse a particular issue in their community; in our project, the sensitive nature of drug use led us to employ a hybrid approach of PhotoVoice and a more individually focused photo-elicitation method.

Clinicians advised the research team that they had developed systems for reminding clients about appointments and events, and suggested that they be involved in helping to recruit clients. We asked the community advisory panel how they wanted to be notified of future research activities and whether they wanted clinicians to be involved. Based on their recommendations and on a case-by-case basis with clients' permission, I (Sarah) provided regular reminders to clients by telephone and in person about research-related appointments. For clients who could not be reached by telephone or email, I asked in advance if reminders could be provided by clinicians or during clinical programmes, like recreation therapy.

While using trusted persons to promote research activities in CBR is common, often those with direct clinical roles are excluded from study recruitment. The team wondered how to balance working with clinicians to decrease barriers to participation while also ensuring that confidentiality was protected. The team also wondered about confidentiality if clinicians took on this role, considering clients would have to indirectly disclose illicit substance use.

This situation raised a number of challenges for us. First, the distinctions between clinical care and research were difficult to navigate. In a hospital environment, clients could not be as anonymous as compared with a community-based setting; clinicians and staff needed to know where they were for their safety and to provide care in the form of medications, specialised meals, etc. As well, clients living in the community had to sign in at the front door and were expected to advise staff of who they were seeing. This issue was difficult to mitigate because we conducted the project at the hospital to ensure location was not a barrier for participation. To resolve this, we advised participants that anyone on the research team in a clinical role at the hospital would only have access to aggregated data. Participants could be either substance users or non-substance users, and so participating in the project would not inadvertently disclose someone's drug use status.

Second, clients often relayed information to me through their clinician and vice versa. When speaking with clients we always stressed that the research was separate from their other hospital-related appointments, but some clients still got confused. We consistently reminded both clients and staff of the nature of the project, and continually asked for clients' permission when sharing information through clinicians. Informed consent was also not a one-time event; rather, we used a multi-staged consent process. This included phone or in-person conversations prior to the actual interview to discuss the nature of the project and any concerns participants might have. Then we checked in with participants after the interview in cases where we were concerned that photographs they shared might compromise anonymity (e.g. photos of participants' homes where they were also seen by clinicians).

Third, as a research coordinator, I had to be very conscious about what information I was sharing and with whom. I shared an office with the recreation therapist, which proved very useful in supporting clients (helping to arrange transportation, scheduling interviews around other appointments, etc.). However, because clinicians were used to sharing information with each other within the hospital, I had to sometimes excuse myself from conversations or be guarded in my responses to questions (e.g., clinicians asking questions about clients' photographs, etc.). Even issues of when I could make telephone calls became challenging both ethically and logistically as I shared office space with a clinician.

The issue of confidentiality and avoiding harm was balanced with clients' desire to participate in research and also their trust in the integrity of the clinical and research team. On-going check-ins with the larger team, regular reflexive note-taking and access to multiple support people (academic researchers and a clinical manager) provided different avenues to reflect and debrief depending on the issue. This case taught us that ethical issues are very particular to context, and research teams are wise to carefully address all of the issues prior to and throughout a CBR project.

Commentary on Case 6.2

Kristin Kalsem

This case study highlights the vigilance necessary to make certain that anonymity, privacy, and confidentiality are maintained on agreed-upon terms. As the researchers point out, they had to continually remind the participants not to inadvertently give information to their clinical providers that would identify them or compromise the confidentiality of the data or their own privacy. It is an excellent example of the fact that 'informed consent' is often not a one-time event.

The relatively small community here also presented challenges, especially with respect to anonymity. Given the context of this study, there were so many ways that anonymity could be lost. Accepting this, the researchers took steps to minimise any negative impacts that could result from compromised anonymity. For example, the researchers made it known that both substance users and non-substance users could participate in the study. In this way, one's participation in the study itself did not disclose this private information. Also, clinicians on the research team only had access to aggregated data which also avoided any issues that might have arisen if they learned, for example, about illicit drug use.

This case study also raises issues of anonymity, privacy, and confidentiality that can arise when a common methodology of PR is used – PhotoVoice. PhotoVoice projects often may include pictures of the participants themselves, their families, homes or other identifying information. Depending on the research question, they also may include pictures that raise sensitive privacy concerns. In this research, anticipating that the sensitive nature of drug use might result in some of these issues, the researchers adapted the PhotoVoice project. It was still necessary, however, to carefully monitor the photographs on an on-going basis.

The fact that PR is community-based and brings a wide variety of expertise to the research team to facilitate the best outcomes is one of its greatest strengths. This case study illustrates, however, that it also may result in a blurring of boundaries (Who is part of the research team? Who on the team has access to what data?) that could be problematic if not carefully monitored. Here, that careful supervision was in place. There was a research coordinator whose explicit responsibilities included taking all steps possible on an ongoing basis to ensure that anonymity, privacy, and confidentiality were maintained.

Case 6.3 Tensions between confidentiality and equitable recognition of co-researchers: Participatory health research in a Swazi village

Michelle Brear

Introduction

This case was written by an Australian academic, undertaking participatory health research in a rural village in Swaziland (now known as eSwatini) for a PhD. The community was physically isolated due to lack of services (especially transport) and socially marginalised by poverty, poor living and agricultural conditions, and challenges accessing important services like health clinics, employment, and schools.

The case

Protecting the confidentiality of research participants (including individuals and entire communities) is a key principle of ethical research conduct. However, in participatory health research (PHR), equitably recognising the contributions of community co-researchers is also an important ethical principle. This case study highlights how these two principles may be in tension, if we believe that equitably recognising co-researchers relies on their identification. Tensions between these two principles arose for me when I was conducting my PhD research.

Before starting my PhD, I had been working voluntarily in a preschool in a village of about 1,000 inhabitants in Swaziland for about five years. I was introduced to the community by a local business person and my voluntary work included helping open and register the preschool at the community's request and working in the classroom alongside a local teacher for the first year of the school's operation. At that time I lived in the community with a family. When I moved to the nearest town to take a paying job, I continued to participate in the preschool as a member of the school committee and by helping the teachers learn to use computers and develop writing skills, and doing fundraising to cover the operating and infrastructure development costs. I decided to do the research for the PhD because I became interested in documenting the process and the challenges the community faced in this grassroots work. I initiated the research project and the preschool teachers and parents agreed to participate. The preschool was the partner organisation. The research was about the state of people's health and how it might be enhanced through a community preschool.

I facilitated community participation in the PHR through a series of experiential learning workshops, in which a group of eight community co-researchers and I co-learnt about research and the community. We co-designed a multiple-methods research study with assistance from senior academic supervisors based in Australia. The community co-researchers later implemented the study in the community (i.e. collected and analysed data and disseminated results).

I was simultaneously collecting ethnographic data about the co-researchers' participation in, and human development through, PHR. The aim of that study was to understand participation and empowerment in the PHR process. I designed and implemented the ethnographic study independently of the co-researchers, who were participants/respondents. However, I applied some PHR principles in the implementation, for example I discussed the results with the co-researchers. I had analysed the ethnographic data about the nature of the 'empowerment' of the community researchers through experiential learning, and prepared the results as a conference poster.

The tension between the ethical principles of confidentiality in human subjects research and recognition of co-researchers in participatory research became apparent in a 'member checking' session, in which I presented the poster and listened to the co-researchers' feedback on it. One of the co-researchers said that he agreed with what I had written about them becoming empowered, but had a small problem. 'It's this pseudonym you're using,' he said. 'It would be better if it was my real name and then everyone would know it was me that did this research.' The other co-researchers agreed with him. One flushed as she spoke of how proud she would feel, having her name on the poster for the world to see and know that she had played an important role in research.

Immediately after hearing these comments, I felt very pleased that the co-researchers wanted to be named. It indicated to me that they had a sense of ownership of the research and had developed self-esteem and considered the work they had done valuable. My only concern was the need to seek further approval from the ethics committees that had approved my research on the condition that confidentiality was protected. I was concerned permission might not be granted by these committees, the members of which likely had no experience of participatory research and were probably unfamiliar with its principle of equitable recognition.

My concerns mounted after speaking to other senior Australian academics who were involved in the project. They advised caution in naming the co-researchers, highlighting that identifying any of them might inadvertently identify the community and other participants in the research, who may want their confidentiality protected. They recommended further discussions with the community, and particularly key informants who might potentially be identified inadvertently. I agreed and asked the co-researchers to wait to identify themselves. They agreed.

In partnership, we organised discussions with individual key informants and at community meetings. At the end of each discussion the individuals and groups provided verbal consent for the co-researchers and the community as a whole to be identified. They thought this was a good approach because unless the community was named, how could the results of the research be used as evidence to support funding applications for future actions?

But I was still concerned. Some of the people who made the decision to identify the community had not been respondents in the research, and others who had been, were not at the meeting. The people we spoke to did not seem to consider in any great depth the potential for negative ramifications to arise from individuals being identified (rather they assumed they would not occur). I also had difficulty thinking of realistic examples of how the identification of the community members might be detrimental, but was concerned that there was potential for unforeseen negative ramifications.

Ultimately the co-researcher participants decided that they wanted me to use pseudonyms in articles in which I presented the results of the ethnography of the process and outcomes of the PHR (in which they were participants). I published these using my real name, with the co-researchers' consent. We have not identified the community by name in articles detailing the results of the ethnography or PHR. However, two of the co-researchers co-authored academic conference and/or journal articles detailing the results of the PHR (in which they were co-researchers). They used their real names, with the agreement of the co-researcher group. To date I am not aware of any adverse consequences for the entire community or individual co-researchers that have occurred as a result of either the co-researchers or me revealing our identities.

Commentary on Case 6.3

Kristin Kalsem

This case illustrates the ethical dilemma of weighing the value of maintaining anonymity, privacy, and confidentiality against the value of acknowledging and giving credit to community co-researchers. It also raises complex and difficult questions regarding the rights of a 'community' as a whole.

As Kaufman and Ramarao note in their overview of research ethics and the implications for communities, 'within the context of the research process, community confidentiality, community risks and benefits, individual autonomy, and individual risks and benefits are interconnected' (2005, p. 156). In this case study, the participants specifically asked to be identified with their real names which indicated to the researcher the pride and sense of ownership that they felt in the research project. This type of empowerment is precisely one of the primary goals of PR. On the other hand, the researcher was concerned that the governing ethics board would not approve disclosing these names because it had approved the project on the condition of anonymity. Also, other academic researchers urged consideration of the community's rights regarding anonymity, privacy, and confidentiality. What if recognising the participants who did give individual consent to being identified inadvertently identified others?

More so than many traditional researchers who take a very individualised approach, participatory researchers long have been thinking in terms of the rights of communities (Banks et al., 2013). Moreover, the relationships to the communities that are developed during the PR process can make it easier to address issues as they arise. In this case study, for example, it was possible to hold community meetings and the community had been sufficiently involved in the research to understand the risks and benefits involved. Community members also seemed very tuned in to the action-orientation of PR in that they identified a benefit of non-anonymity being the ability to apply for future funding.

In the original draft of this case study that was submitted for this publication, the researcher had chosen to act 'safely', complying with agreed-upon measures that resulted in ethics review board approval. She did not identify herself either, listing the author as 'anonymous'. It was clear at that point, however, that the researcher was struggling with whether the decision not to disclose the community co-researchers was also a power issue. Was the academic community with its position and rules getting the final say? The researcher expressed hope that she would be able to fulfil obligations of what Banks et al. identify as 'everyday ethics' in the near future. 'Everyday ethics' emphasise the 'situated nature of ethics, with a focus on qualities of character and responsibilities attaching to particular relationships (as opposed to the articulation and implementation of abstract principles and rules)' (Banks et al., 2013, p. 263). Indeed, as the final version of this case study reveals, steps in that direction have been taken. After further discussions with her co-researchers, arrangements have been made to fit different situations. Pseudonyms for participants have been used in certain contexts; the author and two of her co-researchers have identified themselves in others. The actual process of reflecting on these complex issues has led to more nuanced decision making. At this juncture, the community itself has not been identified. Given the expressed desire of some community members to build on the research to obtain additional funding, however, it seems important to bring these ongoing discussions back to the community, specifically to grapple with the issue of what would constitute community consent.

Case 6.4 Could we protect confidentiality, and for whom? Story from a PhotoVoice project with teenagers living with Autism Spectrum Disorder in Hanoi, Vietnam

Vu Song Ha

Introduction

This case study is contributed by a researcher from Vietnam, based on her experience of carrying out a PhotoVoice project with nine teenagers with Autism Spectrum Disorder (ASD), a life-long neurodevelopment disorder characterised by difficulties in social communication and interaction, and restricted and repetitive patterns of behaviour, in Hanoi, Vietnam from July 2011 to May 2012. This PhotoVoice project is a part of her PhD program at the School of Population Health of the University of Queensland, Australia. Findings from this project and its PhotoVoice exhibition at the end extended understandings of the lived experience of living with ASD in Hanoi, and raised public awareness on ASD. However, some issues emerged from this study, including whether and how to maintain confidentiality when the teenagers are the people who tell about their own lives and educate the broader community through their photos, and who decides if the teenagers should be given pseudonyms or be named, and what the benefits and risks of this decision are for the young people and their families.

The case

At the beginning of this project, I sent information sheets to the parents of teenagers with ASD and sought their informed consent for their children to participate in my study. In the information sheet, I described the purpose and process of the research, benefits, risks, the ownership of photos, confidentiality, and a process for asking permission when taking photos. I also mentioned the opportunity to display visual images to raise public awareness on ASD, and described the process for obtaining separate informed consent for displaying photographs in public at a later date. These topics were all revisited at various times during the PhotoVoice project with the teenagers themselves.

Regarding confidentiality, although I stored photos of the children in folders with their names coded, it did not ensure confidentiality, since a number of the teenagers took photos of themselves (self-portraits) or their family members. I realised that the teenagers felt comfortable taking their own photos and showing them to me. At the same time, while parents whose children were participating in this project were very supportive, a couple of them felt uncomfortable to be shown in photographs taken by their children. One mother covered her face, and another mother told me that even though it was fine to be included in photos taken for research, she did not want photographs with her or her husband's faces to be seen by others.

The PhotoVoice exhibition added to the complexities of insuring confidentiality. These included discussions about how to establish a balance between the ethical principles in research of ensuring confidentiality and the potential benefits of the PhotoVoice exhibition for public education on autism to make change. We also considered what to do with photographs which included recognisable names or faces, and whether the teenagers would be acknowledged as authors of the exhibition. Even though I discussed the risks of disclosing personal identity at the exhibition with the parents, most of the children and parents wanted to use the children's real names in their photographs, only one teenager and her mother chose to use her nickname. Some teenagers used their first names only, while the rest used their full names. The majority of parents provided permission to show all photos that their children selected for exhibition even with their children and their own faces. A couple of parents withdrew photos with their faces. All families were happy to drive their children to attend the opening and surprisingly, the parents designed and printed a special T-shirt for them to wear. It made me a little bit nervous since I worried that the teenagers and other family members might feel that their children were being labeled and disclosed due to a number of members of the media who came to report the event. However, I witnessed that instead of worries, parents showed their pride in their children as the creators of the photographs and key persons at the exhibition. They invited their relatives to come to the exhibition and showed their relatives their children's photographs. In addition, visitors from the media expressed very positive feedback on the exhibition, the teenagers with ASD, and their families.

The PhotoVoice exhibition was good for public awareness raising and advocacy, but it affected the confidentiality of my research. Though I used pseudonyms for the teenagers in the research itself, several parents in the Hanoi Club of parents of children with ASD, who had not participated in the study, knew the children who participated in this study.

In my dissertation I used pseudonyms for all of my participants including teenagers in the PhotoVoice project. When I prepared my paper on this PhotoVoice project for publication in a peer-reviewed journal, I also followed the instruction of the journal to use all pseudonyms for the teenagers, as research participants. It was considered common practice for me as a researcher. However, when I contacted some families again for their permission to use their children's photographs for my paper, they asked me why we needed to use pseudonyms when their children had disclosed their condition, and they (and their teenagers – as they said) would be happy to have their children be recognised with their real names in the paper.

Thus, I wonder in which context the teenagers and their families are more at risk when their real names and identities are disclosed: at the exhibition in their own community, in the media, or in international peer-reviewed journals? I am aware of the need for protection of research participants and their families, and there is a possibility that parents and teenagers might not fully recognise all of the risks of disclosure. Nevertheless, do we always know better than the parents, who have great resilience, and have been creating social movements for the rights of individuals living with ASD? When the teenagers and their parents choose to speak out and become advocates for their needs and rights, is it possible for them to be recognised as change agents and authors rather than research participants who need to be protected?

As a participatory action researcher, this PhotoVoice project provided opportunities for me to learn about the lives of teenagers with ASD, and work with them and their parents as partners to organise the PhotoVoice exhibition as a public awareness raising activity. Though the confidentiality of the teenagers and their family members sometimes could not be protected, I believe that families could make well-informed decisions regarding this aspect of their participation. In addition, we also need to acknowledge that the teenagers and their families are not only vulnerable research participants, but also change agents, and it will be beneficial if they are engaged in the discourse of confidentiality in action research and publication.

Commentary on Case 6.4

Kristin Kalsem

A major goal of this PR project was public education, making people more aware of the realities of living with autism spectrum disorder (ASD). The method chosen by the participants was PhotoVoice and the planned action was a public exhibition of visual images taken by the teenagers with ASD participating in the study. What role should anonymity, privacy, and confidentiality play in a project like this?

The researcher approached this issue very thoughtfully, providing detailed information to the teenagers and their parents at the outset when obtaining their informed consent to participate in the study. Recognising that participants may have different anonymity, privacy, and confidentiality concerns in different contexts, she also prepared a separate consent for the public display. It also is clear that she spent much time developing trust with the participants and their parents in that they felt comfortable approaching her when they had concerns or wanted to limit access to personal information. Flexibility in the design of the project allowed participants to participate with different levels of disclosure of identifying information.

It is telling that, when it came to the academic part of the project, the researcher (as I would have) automatically complied with the 'common practice' of using pseudonyms. It was the participants who questioned that traditional rule and gave insight into the different value of giving credit and public voice to persons who are not usually acknowledged for their contributions in academic research. Brydon-Miller and Greenwood in their reflections on the dissonance between traditional ethics research practises and central tenets of PR ask: 'When does protection become paternalism, and concern become control?' (2006, p. 122). In this case study, the researcher who *knows* the participants and their parents feels confident that they can make informed decisions for themselves and reminds us that, as participants in PR, they are change agents who deserve to have their say.

PART 3: CONCLUDING COMMENTS

Kristin Kalsem

In reviewing the literature on PR and anonymity, privacy, and confidentiality, as well as reading case studies in the scholarship and included in this chapter, I was struck by the obvious: the key to successful outcomes and the crux of suggested best practises is – participation. Fundamental to PR is the belief that stakeholders must be involved in meaningful research and problem-solving. Issues of anonymity, privacy, and confidentiality must be addressed in all research. Thus, it only makes sense to have co-researchers and other members of a community as involved as possible in these issues too. In each of the examples in this chapter, co-researchers and participants helped to address various issues that arose in the course of the research. But, as also was discussed, there is room to expand participation such that participants are involved *before* there are issues to address. This means including concerns relating to anonymity, privacy, and confidentiality in the research training. This means involving co-researchers in drafting informed consent forms. This in turn means, to the extent possible, including co-researchers and other participants in the ethics review board process itself. Sometimes, anonymity, privacy, and confidentiality must be maintained for important reasons. Other times, there may be value in making exceptions. As in all other aspects of research, co-researchers and other community participants have important insights and perspectives to offer. Their contributions can help educate ethics review boards about the process, benefits, and value of PR.

References

Banks, S., Armstrong, A., Carter, K., Graham, H., Hayward, P., Henry, A., Holland, T., Holmes, C., Lee, A., McNulty, A., Moore, N., Nayling, N., Stokoe, A. & Strachan, A. (2013). Everyday ethics in community-based participatory research. *Contemporary Social Science, 8*(3), 263–277.

Bradley, M. (2007). Silenced for their own protection: How the IRB marginalizes those it feigns to protect. *ACME: An International E-Journal for Critical Geographies, 6*(3), 339–349.

Brydon-Miller, M. & Greenwood, D. (2006). A re-examination of the relationship between action research and human subjects review processes. *Action Research, 4*(1), 117–128.

Easter, M., Davis, A. & Henderson, G. (2004). Confidentiality: More than a linkage file and a locked drawer. *IRB: Ethics & Human Research, 26*(2), 13–17.

Kaufman, C. & Ramarao, S. (2005). Community confidentiality, consent, and the individual research process: Implications for demographic research. *Population Research and Policy Review, 24*(2), 149–173.

Lincoln, Y. & Guba, E. (1989). Ethics: The failure of positive science. *Review of Higher Education, 12*(3), 221–240.

Merritt, M., Labrique, A., Katz, J., Mahbubur, R., West, K. & Pettit, J. (2010). A field training guide for human subjects research ethics. *PLoS Medicine, 7*(10), 1–4.

Morse, J. (1998). The contractual relationship: Ensuring protection of anonymity and confidentiality. *Qualitative Health Research, 8*(3), 301–303.

Parent, W. A. (1983). Privacy, morality, and the law. *Philosophy & Public Affairs, 12*(4), 269–288.

Pritchard, I. (2002). Travelers and trolls: Practitioner research and institutional review boards. *Educational Researcher, 31*(3), 3–13.

Stuart, C. (1998). Care and concern: An ethical journey in participatory action research. *Canadian Journal of Counseling, 32*(4), 298–314.

van den Hoonaard, W. (2003). Is anonymity an artifact in ethnographic research? *Journal of Academic Ethics, 1*(2), 141–151.

Wiles, R., Charles, V., Crow, G. & Heath, S. (2006). Researching researchers: Lessons for research ethics. *Qualitative Research, 6*(3), 283–299.

Yanar, Z., Fazli, M., Rahman, J. & Farthing, R. (2016). Research ethics committees and participatory action research with young people: The politics of voice. *Journal of Empirical Research on Human Research Ethics, 11*(2), 122–128.

7

INSTITUTIONAL ETHICAL REVIEW PROCESSES

Adrian Guta

With cases contributed by Colin Bradley, Anne MacFarlane, Jane Jervis, Geralyn Hynes, and Jon Fieldhouse

PART 1: INTRODUCTION AND OVERVIEW OF ISSUES

Adrian Guta

Background

The participatory research literature identifies navigating institutional ethical review and obtaining approval as potentially challenging. These challenges are attributed to the biomedical and positivist standards used by most institutional ethical review boards (Guillemin & Gillam, 2004). While many of the assumptions underlying the ethical review process are problematic for all social research, they pose specific challenges for participatory research. Ethical guidelines for research and institutional forms are often premised on a clear distinction between researchers and subjects of research, and the relational and flexible nature of participatory studies may be surprising to ethical review boards. This chapter introduction will provide an overview of key debates in the literature but also highlights emerging examples of researchers and review boards working together. First, I will locate myself in this discourse and provide an overview of the tensions between traditional and participatory conceptions of research ethics. Then I will offer insights from my own experiences as a participatory researcher and ethical review board member. In Part 2, four cases provided by different participatory researchers and teams will be presented, each exploring a different challenge encountered when obtaining ethical review. I will offer short reflective commentaries on each case, before giving some concluding comments in Part 3.

Before delving further, I wish to locate myself as someone with training in social work, public health, and bioethics. I have been involved in various research projects using community-based, participatory, and action elements for over a decade in Canada. These studies explored the needs of people living with or at risk of acquiring HIV, and had elements of sexuality, substance use, sex work, illness, and other issues often deemed sensitive. The first of these was my work with the Toronto Teen Survey Team where we made a social justice argument about the importance of allowing adolescents as young as 13 years old to participate in research about sexual health without obtaining parental consent (Flicker & Guta, 2008). More recently, I have been involved in research which has brought participatory approaches into a hospital to engage people living with HIV and who use substances in collaborative arts-based research (Strike et al., 2016; Switzer et al., 2015). I have experience submitting research on sensitive topics using unconventional methods to ethical review boards. I also served for over a decade on ethical review boards and reviewed protocols using a range of community-engaged and traditional approaches. In my capacity as a reviewer, I was often struck by the lack of detail in submissions, including those claiming to be participatory. Finally, I have researched the experiences of participatory researchers and ethical review board stakeholders about their respective experiences (Flicker et al., 2015; Guta et al., 2016; Guta et al., 2012; Guta, Nixon, et al., 2013; Guta, Wilson et al., 2010). As such, I attempt to take a balanced approach to discussing the role of ethical review for participatory research. However, my primary concern is always the protection of research participants.

The research ethics review process

The requirement to submit research for pre-review to an independent committee emerged in reaction to the egregious historical acts committed against human subjects in the name of 'science' (Chadwick, 1997; Jones, 1993; Reverby, 2009; Rothman, 1982). The Nazi eugenics experiments (Grodin & Annas, 1996), Tuskegee syphilis study (Freimuth et al., 2001), the Willowbrook State School hepatitis study (Krugman, 1986) and others, resulted in the development of national and international codes to protect human rights. These include the Nuremberg Code (1949), the Declaration of Helsinki (World Medical Association Declaration of Helsinki, 1964), and the Belmont Report (Office of Secretary, 1979). These protections were further informed by questionable social science research which introduced new forms of emotional and social harms (Babbie, 2004; Humphreys, 1970; Milgram, 1974; Zimbardo, 1973). Collectively, these protections recognise the dignity of human life, require consent from human research subjects or 'participants', and permit consent to be withdrawn. These initial protections have evolved into 'over 1,000 laws, regulations, and guidelines on human subjects protections' (International Compilation of Human Research Protections, 2017). The requirements for a formal independent ethical review are enforced differently around the world with individual countries having various degrees of research ethics infrastructure and legal requirements.

In response to the growth of what has been termed a 'research ethics industry' (Allen, 2008; Ashcroft, 1999), researchers are questioning whether ethical review boards are effective and accountable (Coleman & Bouesseau, 2008; Savulescu, Chalmers, & Blunt, 1996), and whether they do anything besides 'checking off boxes' (Ashcroft & Pfeffer, 2001; O'Reilly et al., 2009). Others in the academy have gone as far as to claim ethical review constitutes a threat to academic freedom (Dingwall, 2008; Haggerty, 2004; Lewis, 2008). The term 'ethics creep', coined by Haggerty (2004), describes a process where ethics review is expanding and colonising aspects of research previously outside of its purview. I am aware of these critiques, but side with Upshur (2011) who points out that ethics review is no different than other forms of peer review researchers must undergo. I have argued that many of the faults in the system are a result of decreasing investment in ethical review at the university level evident in staffing cuts which reduces personalised ethics consultation (Guta, Nixon, et al., 2013). As well, there is the issue of institutional and departmental cultures within some institutions, reflected in their ethical review boards, and researchers may find themselves subject to reviews at socially conservative and risk-averse institutions. As well, much has been written about the challenges experienced by researchers who must obtain multi-site reviews which are often contradictory (Green et al., 2006).

An issue requiring some discussion is the tension which emerges between conceptions of research ethics, rooted in a positivistic bio-medical approach to research, and participatory approaches rooted in collaboration, shared decision-making, and co-ownership. The ongoing critique is that ethical review imposes a biomedical conception of harm, vulnerability, and autonomy (Hoeyer, 2006; Hoeyer et al., 2005). Within biomedical research, risks are understood as knowable, discreet and manageable, like the conditions in an experiment. Risks are mitigated through techniques such as minimal contact between researcher and subject and fixed research procedures (e.g. the intervention will be administered the same way each time). Such specificity is easily transferred from a research proposal to an ethics protocol. However, this creates challenges for participatory approaches which are flexible and evolve throughout the project. Early on in this debate Downie and Cottrell (2001) argued that ethical review boards are not equipped to deal with the kinds of 'non-traditional' methods used in participatory research; the process is 'frustrating and sometimes demoralizing' (p. 9), takes too long, and fails to address ongoing ethical issues. Overall, the literature contrasts the bureaucratic nature of ethical review with the emancipatory goals of participatory research (Blake, 2007; Boser, 2006, 2007; Martin, 2007; Rolfe, 2005; Shore, 2006). As participatory approaches have gained popularity, some ethical review boards have improved their processes by adding options for participatory research on their forms alongside biomedical research (acknowledging this is a legitimate research approach). Others have taken it a step further by providing board members and staff education about participatory approaches and inviting researchers to meetings to discuss their work (Guta et al., 2012; Guta, Wilson, et al., 2010). Finally, boards are taking steps to ensure they have members with appropriate expertise to review participatory research.

Wolf (2010) has pointed out there may be misunderstanding and confusion on both sides of the review which requires discussion and education. In the following section, I will describe some common points of tension identified in the participatory ethics literature, and from my personal experience wearing two hats (participatory researcher and ethical review board member). Before comparing both groups as if they are distinct, it is critical to point out that participatory researchers and ethical review board members have a shared interest in protecting research participants and ensuring research is conducted in an ethical manner. This is of central importance and should guide all discussions. Common points of shared interest are the rationale for the study, conflicts of interest, research methodology, participants and related risks and benefits, informed consent, and privacy and confidentiality. These are issues of interest to both ethical review boards and participatory researchers and about which they strive to maintain high standards. However, many participatory scholars would expand these criteria beyond individual protections to account for the community level risks and benefits (Flicker et al., 2007) and for the relational and everyday ethical issues that arise in the practice of participatory research (Banks et al., 2013; Guta et al., 2016). I will explore some of the key issues which arise during the ethical review process below, with a focus on how ethical review boards may interpret them in relation to participatory research and how researchers can respond. It is outside the scope of this chapter to explore all ethical issues in participatory research, and many issues are discussed in other chapters.

Conflicts of interest

One of the first sections of most ethical review forms asks about potential conflicts of interest (e.g., if the researcher has a previous relationship with participants or stands to benefit from the research). Ethical review boards expect a clear separation between those who could be perceived to have a conflict of interest and the research process. Indeed, the ideal situation is a disinterested party conducting the research. However, this is not the reality of participatory research where members of research teams are often directly affected by the research and may have various roles: researcher, service provider, clinician, volunteer, member of the Board of Directors, client/patient/service user, etc. The direct involvement of those most affected and the diversity of perspectives is understood to improve research but may raise concerns for ethical review boards. Research teams will need to explain the different roles of team members and identify where potential conflicts exist (although they may not see them as conflicts per se). It may be helpful to provide the ethical review board with some terms of reference or memorandum of understanding that will outline roles, responsibilities, and decision-making structures in the project. Participatory research teams will need to develop protections to prevent conflicts of interest from influencing the research. This *may* require members of the research team with dual roles (e.g., a member of the research team who also provides direct services to potential participants, or a researcher who also sits on the Board of Directors of a partnering organisation) to take a step back from the project at times and have minimal involvement in tasks like data collection. In my work with clinicians and service providers, they understood the need for these protections and were happy to be brought back into the project during the data analysis phase to review anonymised aggregated data. However, when working in a participatory manner such a separation may not always be necessary or welcome. Ethical review boards may assume that dual roles are inherently coercive, but participants may welcome or even expect trusted figures to approach them. For example, the service provider who is also a researcher may be one of the few trusted sources within a community and members of that community may be unwilling to share their information with any other interviewer. Research teams are encouraged to consider the pros and cons of such an approach and explain their rationale to an ethical review board.

Peer researchers

Peer researchers are members of a community who research aspects of the lives of their peers (Flicker, Guta, et al., 2010; Greene et al., 2009). An example might be young researchers studying the leisure pursuits of other young people living in the same neighbourhood. In some projects, peer researchers partner in all facets of a research project and take on a leadership role. In other projects, their role is more instrumental and they are involved in key aspects of the research (e.g., participant recruitment and data collection). The close involvement of community members in this way has raised questions about whether they can maintain ethical standards when working in their communities (Bean & Silva, 2010; Constantine, 2010; Simon & Mosavel, 2010). Being part of the community is what makes peer researchers excellent recruiters and data collectors but this can put them into uncomfortable situations when they take on a researcher identity (Guta, Flicker, & Roche, 2013; Logie et al., 2012). As well, ethical review boards may become confused about the difference between peer researchers and participants if this is not clearly described, and they should be distinguished as members of the research team or as project staff to prevent confusion. Any methods and ethics training they will receive should be noted. The ethical review board may want to know what protections are in place to help peers create boundaries between their social life and the research (e.g., peers do not collect data from anyone they know personally). Research teams should consider how they will integrate, train, and support peer researchers throughout the process (Flicker, Roche, & Guta, 2010; Guta, Flicker, & Roche, 2010; Roche et al., 2010).

Methods

Participatory research has been a testing ground for innovative research designs and new methods. These include mixing methods (qualitative, quantitative, etc.), using arts-based approaches, developing new sampling and recruitment techniques, and the direct involvement of community members. For research teams, this often reflects a desire to maximise inclusion and to collect different kinds of data to support community change. One method may lead into another (e.g., photographs in phase one will inform the focus groups in phase two which will inform the survey in phase three). However, it can be challenging for ethical review boards to stay on top of these developments. While it is outside of the scope of this chapter to discuss all possible methods or their combination, research teams should consider how each additional data collection approach introduces new levels of risk and opportunities for participants to become identifiable. They will need to discuss each of the methods individually and then the implications of bringing them together in one project. Research teams should explain the rationale, and especially if it is rooted in community preferences, for using such a design. Finally, it is not uncommon for research teams to submit reviews that are incomplete (we do not know what phase two will look like until we have completed phase one) and expect the ethical review boards to sign off. Research teams should discuss the best way to approach staggered projects with their institutions and for ethical review committees before submitting. Some boards are willing to sign off on work in progress with the condition that an amendment is submitted when the details are finalised, but others would prefer a separate review for each phase. Research teams should explore their options before submitting.

Participants

Ethical review boards want to know who will be participating in the research and why they have been chosen. These questions serve two purposes; the board wants to make sure researchers are not excluding groups of people from the research process because of their characteristics, and to establish if the participants have any pre-existing vulnerability that may prevent them from giving free and informed consent. Most ethical review boards include groups under a protected category, such as pregnant women, prisoners, children and youth below the age of majority, or anyone with cognitive impairments. Researchers may need to establish additional protections to support vulnerable participants. The participant section of the ethics protocol requires researchers to describe their participants' demographic characteristics (age, sex, ethnicity, etc.), their possible vulnerabilities and related risks and benefits from participating in the research, and what protections will be put in place by the research team. Participatory research tends to focus on individuals that are considered vulnerable by ethical review boards because of their social location or individual characteristics. Participatory researchers should not shy away from discussing the vulnerability of the communities they work with. Rather, researchers are advised to use the participants' section to demonstrate a strong understanding of the relevant vulnerabilities and the team's experience and how community knowledge has informed the process. As well, researchers may wish to highlight the experiences of other research teams working with similar populations. In my experience, ethical review boards can be swayed by evidence from the literature. Participatory scholarship has arguably gone 'mainstream' (Horowitz et al., 2009) and many teams have written about their experiences (Marshall et al., 2012; Morgan et al., 2014), and how they worked with their ethical review boards

(Chabot et al., 2012; Solomon & Piechowski, 2011). As well, some communities have produced their own guidelines on best practice when researching with them (Jürgens, 2005). What is less convincing are appeals to trust the researcher because they *know* the community. There is no best approach, and even projects which have undertaken consultation with community leaders may find themselves poorly prepared when engaging the larger community.

Recruitment

Ethical review boards will want to know how participants will be recruited (e.g., advertised to potential participants). Recruitment strategies range from putting up a poster explaining the details of the project in a community space and letting participants follow up with the researcher to identifying and approaching participants directly. During recruitment, researchers are usually expected to identify themselves and their institution, the main purpose of the study and the methods, potential risks and benefits, funding sources, any inclusion/exclusion criteria, and what steps are required to participate. Materials should be written at a level appropriate for the participants and technical terms or research jargon should be avoided. The ethical review board will expect to see all recruitment materials – posters, advertisements, flyers, letters, e-mail text, or telephone scripts – to be used for recruitment. Ethical review boards are often very strict with the wording of recruitment materials and require that specific language be used. This is to prevent participants from being provided with different information about the research.

Two issues that participatory research teams are advised to consider include the content of the recruitment materials and who is involved in the recruitment process. First, research teams may want to deviate from standard wording to use community relevant language and images, especially when the research may be stigmatising (e.g., using slang for certain kinds of sexual acts or drug use). Researchers are advised to explain why such wording is more appropriate (e.g., a community advisory board has recommended it). As well, the strategies of having service providers or members of the community recruit raises the potential that participants will feel obliged to participate. In some communities, there may be an expectation that an invitation to participate comes from a trusted person. For teams working with 'hard to reach communities' this approach may be necessary. The ethical review board will need to see that your team has considered the range of recruitment options and that based on consultation with your team/partner agency/advisory committee has decided on the proposed recruitment strategy. As well, the research needs to be differentiated from other services or programmes if relevant. It is advisable to include in the recruitment materials a disclaimer indicating: 'Organization X is a partner on the research but your participation will not affect your current or future access to services.' Ideally, the individual recruiting will not be collecting data and is simply letting potential participants know about the study (they will not benefit or be penalised if anyone participates). However, sometimes community members will opt for unconventional recruitment approaches. This happened in a research project in which I was involved where community members requested their trusted care providers be involved in sending them reminders about the research, as they do with other appointments (see Case 6.2). We explained this to our ethical review board in detail, including why conventional recruitment would not work, and what protections we had in place (e.g., those providing reminders were not part of the research team and would not know who ultimately participated) and they approved our request.

Informed consent process

Ethical review boards are especially concerned about the informed consent process and ensuring participants are given as much information as possible about the research. Traditionally this information is provided in writing and is signed by the participant. A consent form usually identifies the researcher and their home institution; the funding agency if there is one; the purpose of the research; procedures and potential risks and benefits; compensation offered; and a way to contact the ethical review board. These forms should be written in clear and accessible language designed for someone without a scientific background. However, obtaining consent is more than getting a form signed. Consent is an ongoing negotiation between the researcher and participant(s) and may reflect histories of oppression. Some researchers have expressed discomfort over the requirement to use a written document resembling a contract, believing it negatively influences their dynamic with the participant. Participants may feel threatened by a legalistic looking document and feel uncomfortable (e.g., persons in conflict with the law being asked to speak about criminalised activities). Further to this, whole communities may take issue with the requirements for signed consent forms because of how researchers have treated them in the past. For example, much has been written about consent for Indigenous peoples in the context of colonisation and highly unethical behaviour by researchers (Fitzpatrick et al., 2016).

A growing number of ethical review boards are recognising that there are circumstances where a signed consent form is not ideal and may introduce more risk (e.g. asking LGBT youth to get parental consent to participate in research) (Flicker & Guta, 2008). However, research teams are advised to explain what they propose to do in place of signed consent and give details of: 1) why signed consent may be harmful and increase risks associated with participating (e.g. if the forms were subpoenaed); 2) why verbal consent is appropriate and how it will be obtained; and 3) possibly provide examples of other studies where a verbal consent approach was used successfully. This is far more compelling than saying 'having to get signed consent forms will make it harder to get participants' or 'signed consent forms are not culturally appropriate'. Ethical review boards are not concerned with the researcher's timeline or vague appeals to culture, and this should never come before adequately protecting participants. Regardless of whether a written or verbal process is used, researchers should be cognisant of literacy and comprehension issues which may affect the communities with which they work. Researchers need to demonstrate that they have considered the pros and cons of various approaches for obtaining informed consent that are rooted in the communities' needs.

A further consideration for participatory scholars is the role of organisational or community consent. If the researcher is in the organisation in an open way, as may be the case when trying to understand how services are provided, then an organisational consent may be helpful to assure that employees' and clients' interests will be protected. These forms may include a disclaimer that while management is aware of the research and supports it, employees and clients do not have to participate, and are not at risk of losing their jobs or access to services. Researchers who have obtained community consent, for example when working with Indigenous communities, will also need to communicate to participants that the research has been vetted through formal/informal leadership, but that individuals are not obligated to participate. Community consent is not a proxy for individual consent. Researchers should not assume that participants understand this distinction and should remind them of their right to withdraw.

Confidentiality and data management

Ethical review boards want to know how data will be treated after it has been collected and any limitations to maintaining participants' confidentiality (see Chapter 6 for a more detailed discussion of confidentiality). Researchers are required to provide details about how all data (written records, video/audio recordings, artefacts and questionnaires) will be secured. Individual ethical review boards and research institutions may have their own data management requirements. Usually data will be destroyed once it is no longer needed (e.g. interviews will be erased after they are transcribed). These expectations are true of all research, but participatory research may challenge assumptions that participants want their data treated as confidential or that data should be destroyed. Participatory research is often conducted in small communities with close networks. Members of close-knit communities, who use the same services, and see each other regularly, may have different understandings of what is private and what is public. This does not mean researchers would intentionally share information obtained during data collection, but it can be difficult to differentiate what was said where and when. Researchers should be conscious of such barriers to confidentiality, and participants' preferences, when submitting to the ethical review board. The social justice goals of participatory research often result in participants wanting to be identified. Identifying participants, if they choose, can be an excellent way to honour their contribution. However, research teams should not assume participants want to be identified. Participants need to be made aware that information which is shared in a research project may become accessible to people outside of the community.

As well, it may be difficult to maintain the confidentiality of a community with unique attributes and needs. Whereas individual confidentiality can be secured through basic precautions, community confidentiality may be more difficult to secure. Communities may become identifiable by virtue of the researchers involved and through a process of elimination when basic information is provided about a partnering organisation. Research teams should consider how data will reflect onto the larger community and possible implications. For example, could findings from the study be used to further stigmatise participants by those who do not understand the social conditions which may lead to certain behaviours (e.g., the social and legal conditions which lead to high risk drug injection practices)? This does not mean researchers should avoid asking about such issues, especially when the goal is to improve conditions, but that there is an ethical duty related to the framing and dissemination of such information (Flicker et al., 2007). In some of my own research, we have had conversations about the potential for stigmatising the community while balancing the importance of identifying the community partner as a way of honouring the knowledge they provided and their commitment to improving conditions for their clients.

Finally, honouring the knowledge provided by a community may mean returning the data to the community or to individual participants instead of destroying it. This is common when working with Indigenous communities in the Canadian context who have expressly stated that they wish to retain ownership, control, access, and possession (OCAP) over data collected from them (Flicker et al., 2007). This may raise red flags for ethical review boards who expect the data to be destroyed. Researchers should detail why it is important to return the data (e.g., if it has archival or cultural value) and how protections will be put in place to remove individual identifiers or obtain the consent of individual participants to be named, or how the community will be stewarding the data and ensuring it is protected. Whatever the approach to be taken, researchers are asked to provide a detailed justification and data storage or stewardship plan. Individual researchers may still be expected to delete some data from their own records. Overall, participatory forms of research include traditional and emerging issues related to confidentiality. Some participatory projects will include standard interviews and surveys which will be destroyed after use, whereas others may include the collection or development of media (recordings, photos, film) with special meaning. Participatory researchers are often required to push the boundaries between research and community development in ways that challenge and expand traditional ethics.

In the next Part of this chapter, four examples of participatory researchers working with their ethical review committees are presented and discussed. I will offer a brief commentary on each case, reflect on what transpired, and offer suggestions.

PART 2: CASES AND COMMENTARIES

Case 7.1 Approving a participatory research proposal: Perspectives from a Research Ethics Committee Chair and a researcher in Ireland

Colin Bradley and Anne MacFarlane

Introduction

This case concerns a participatory health research project that was submitted for approval to a Research Ethics Committee in Ireland. All researchers wishing to undertake research linked to general medical practice need to submit an application to the Ethics Committee outlining the aims, design and methods, including how people will give consent to participate, how anonymity will be dealt with, potential harm and risk minimised, etc. The case is in two parts. The first part was contributed by a medical academic, based on a time when he chaired the Irish College of General Practitioners Research Ethics Committee. He outlines the Committee's response to an application for approval for a participatory research project. The second part is a short reflection by a health care academic, who was part of the team that submitted the application.

The case

Part 1: Perspectives from the Chair of the Research Ethics Committee

In November 2010, while I was Chair of the Research Ethics Committee of the Irish College of General Practitioners, we received an application for a project entitled 'RESTORE: REsearch into implementation STrategies to support patients of different ORigins and language background in a variety of European primary care settings'. It was quite different from the kind of research proposals we were used to. The committee mostly deals with small investigator led projects from GPs or their trainees who, typically, want to survey patients or their colleagues (using questionnaires or interviews) about various health related issues. We also receive occasional applications from GPs who are involved in trials (primarily post-marketing drug trials) for pharmaceutical companies. The RESTORE project application was for the Irish component of a huge European study regarding how to improve the health care of migrants. It was replete with concepts and language with which the committee was unfamiliar. We were used to randomised controlled designs, cohort studies and descriptive studies. This study was going to use a participatory approach and would involve action research and co-design with stakeholders. This was all very new to us and it was somewhat difficult for us to grasp what exactly all these terms meant. More troubling to us, though, was the paucity of information on exactly who was going to participate in the study and what precisely was the 'intervention'.

We understood that migrants would be involved in the study. We recognised these immediately as a vulnerable group and so we wanted to know how they would be recruited. We wanted to know the sample size and to see the interview schedule. We wanted to know which 'stakeholders' were involved and how they were to be selected. How would informed consent be obtained? What did they mean by migrants 'co-producing' the research? Surely, they are research subjects and need to be protected by standard ethical procedures of being provided detailed participant information and giving informed consent. How can they be researchers and the researched at the same time? The proposal mentioned information being provided in the different languages of the migrants – What languages? What migrant groups? This was all a bit too vague for us to feel our usual degree of comfort.

In the end, we recognised that we had to trust the integrity and expertise of the research group. We came to realise that the very fact of using a participatory approach showed a high degree of sensitivity to the vulnerability of the group that was the focus of the research. We also had to accept that not all the information we were used to having at the outset of a study would be available until the study group commenced their work. We did ask for some clarification of the methods of partic111ipant recruitment and we sought some assurance about the availability of translators/ cultural mediators. We asked that the participant information be simplified. It was a bit too jargonistic even for us, never mind for potential research participants. We wanted to ascertain the burden of time and effort that participation would impose on the participants although, ultimately, we had to accept that this could not be predetermined either. It would really be up to participants themselves, in the end, to judge how much they wanted to put into the research. This was a steep learning curve for both the committee and the researchers. I feel the researchers have come to recognise that a clinical research ethics committee can struggle with the philosophy and methodology of participatory research and that this methodology needs to be described more clearly in language the committee can understand. The committee has also learnt that there is an entirely different approach to research on health and social issues now emerging that is based on very different concepts of research design and a radically different philosophy. They have also come to appreciate that, sometimes, they have to trust that the researchers share the committee's concern for the protection of research 'subjects'. In participatory research this concern is manifest through the 'subjects' being co-designers and co-producers of the research. They are inherently protected from exploitation by the research methodology itself. This being the case, the role of the research ethics committee becomes somewhat less clear. However, there are ethical issues in undertaking participatory research which researchers and ethics committees still need to tease out and learn how to deal with. Perhaps this is something that could be explored in a participatory research project!

Part 2: Reflections from the researcher perspective

I was the lead investigator for this project. The two key learning points for us researchers were that:

1) No matter how much we think we are making complex concepts about participatory research clear, it is likely that we will have to try harder!

2) It was really valuable to say very explicitly in the subsequent ethics applications for this project when and where co-researchers informed the decision making. For example, the recruitment strategy in the RESTORE project has been co-designed with migrants who were community partners in the project. It was important and helpful for the ethics committee members to know that the suggested strategies were considered acceptable by them for their wider community. Furthermore, this also highlighted resilience and expertise among migrants to balance out the inevitable concerns of the ethics committee about their potential vulnerability.

Commentary on Case 7.1

Adrian Guta

This case highlights what it is like to be on opposite sides of the review and the considerations for both the ethical review board and the researcher. From the review board side, I am sympathetic to the need for more information about the research project. Regardless of the approach taken, whether a clinical trial or a participatory project, researchers should be as clear as possible about what they are doing. While researchers would like to have reviewers who are knowledgable about their approach, they should speak to as broad an audience as possible. From the researchers' side, it appears that some additional information, including details about how the community was involved in the decision-making process swayed the ethical review board into approving their protocol. In all, this sounds like a productive exchange between the two groups.

However, I would like to add a word of caution about the claim that participants 'are inherently protected from exploitation by the research methodology itself'. In this case it is coming from an ethical review board, but I have usually heard it coming from participatory researchers. I would respectfully question this, as someone experienced in participatory approaches. While there may be protections from some harms, others are likely to emerge, and the risk of exploitation is always present. As participatory approaches have expanded, and in some cases become a requirement, the risk of unprepared researchers using these approaches has grown. Ethical review boards need to be vigilant to protect communities from those who would claim to have their best interests in mind. This may include challenging claims by so-called community leaders who may not represent the community at large.

Case 7.2 The question of parental consent for teenagers in a doctoral research project in the UK

Jane Jervis

Introduction

This case is provided by a part-time PhD student, conducting research in the United Kingdom (UK). The student was an Advanced Nurse Practitioner (ANP) with a 20-year history of working in the National Health Service (NHS) and on the topic of the PhD related to children visiting ill adult relatives in any hospital ward or department. In clinical practice children were regularly wanting to visit acutely ill or dying relatives, which caused debate with nursing and medical colleagues concerned that they had very limited (or no) knowledge and experience of dealing with children in this type of situation, and that there was no guidance available within hospital policy.

The case

The initial aim of the research study was to use participatory action research (PAR) to identify and critically explore the issues; increase understanding of how staff could be better prepared to support families with children; and to explore the feasibility for staff to improve the quality of service provided. PAR was the framework of choice as it met the requirements of the research questions, aims and core issues while engendering flexibility and inclusion throughout. Prior to the research proposal, consultation focus groups were held with two groups of children and young people (N = 23) from the Medicines for Children Research Network (MCRN). They were asked their opinions on the importance of the research proposed and whether children should (or could) be involved and this feedback contributed to the research design.

The research was planned in two phases. In Phase One Registered Nurses participated in focus groups which identified and explored the issues involved when children or young people visited acutely ill relatives at the hospital; and strategies which could be used to address these issues. Stakeholders identified during the focus groups in Phase One were contacted directly by the researcher by e-mail or verbally and invited to participate in Phase Two of the project.

Currently, any research in the UK involving human participants, human tissue, or personal information must be approved by an independent recognised research ethics committee. If the research proposal involves patients or users of the NHS then it must gain ethical approval from an appropriate National Health Service (NHS) Research Ethics Committee (REC). This was not required for my research as it involved NHS staff and as such did not require NHS REC approval. Since it involved human subjects/participation approval from the University's Ethical Review Panel (ERP) was required and granted; as was permission for the research by the Research and Development Department (R&D) of the relevant hospital.

Phase One generated ideas for strategies to improve the care provided to young people visiting the hospital which required collaboration from stakeholders, such as hospital management and the local children's hospice. For example, one recommendation related to the availability of appropriate resources, such as guidance leaflets and internet information for parents and young people. The hospital had a widening participation programme with local schools and colleges and the co-ordinator had seen and shared the research invitation with them. The researcher was approached by student representatives from one college expressing an interest in participating in the research. The students, aged between 16 and 20 years, were interested in designing resources, and participating in a focus group to reflect upon their work within the study providing a young person's perspective.

In collaboration with college tutors it was decided that the focus groups could take place at the college to ensure a safe and comfortable environment for the students. A familiar tutor could attend to provide support and, as there was a possibility that personal discussions about visiting acutely ill relatives may occur, the risk of anxiety and distress if recounting painful memories was recognised. A counselling service was available at the college as well as Learner Managers who support students with all of their holistic needs. Access to the college support service for the participants was agreed in advance of the Focus Groups.

Although the participation of young people in the project was an exciting proposition and would add a valuable perspective, it did leave me with an ethical dilemma: could the students consent themselves to take part in the research? To enable student participation the researcher applied for an amendment to the original Research Ethical Review Panel approval to request that parental consent not be required for these participants. The main question was whether parental consent was needed or not? Following the submitted amendment, the ERP wrote back requesting detailed information about why parental consent was not being sought.

It was decided that since the students involved had left school, were now at college studying a Level 3 qualification and hoping to go into health care or teaching careers, parental consent was not necessary. All of the students regularly gave their own consent for other college business and the college tutors thought that asking for parental consent may alienate the students. When the research had first come to the student's attention they had made the decision to participate and the aim was to actively involve them as partners as opposed to subjects of the research. It was concerning that asking for parental consent of people who could legally consent to other things (for example, sexual activity) could affect the balance of power between researcher and participants. The literature regarding involving young people in research supported this decision. This was not a situation in which the literature advocated parental consent, such as conducting an interview with a young person under the age of 18 in the family home, vulnerable 16–18 year olds (for example if they had an intellectual disability), or related to an exceptionally sensitive or troubling topic. After providing this information to the ERP, the amendment was subsequently approved and the involvement of the college students commenced. During the focus group the young people stated that they frequently felt patronised and disenfranchised; pursuing parental consent in this age group in this research study could have further compounded this perspective.

Commentary on Case 7.2

Adrian Guta

This case offers an example of a team of researchers requesting to deviate from an ethical review board's recommendations by not obtaining parental consent. In this case, the researchers offered a well-reasoned explanation about why they were deviating from the requirement to obtain parental consent and what protections they had put in place in the form of counselling support for the young people involved. It is highly relevant that participants were being asked for parental consent to participate in research of this nature, but were deemed competent to consent to other higher risk activities. Indeed, those same youth would likely have been able to consent to care in the hospital where the research was to be conducted. As well, the researchers demonstrate an understanding of the ethics literature which does not suggest this is an inherently vulnerable group, and they argue as to why these youth demonstrate a high degree of personal agency and decision-making capacity. The requirement to obtain parental consent for youth in the range of 16–20 years highlights the differences between ethical review boards in different jurisdictions about who can provide free and informed consent. In the Canadian context, 16-year-olds are regularly included in research without parental consent whereas in the United States various laws and regulations require persons as old as 21 to provide parental consent and require researchers to obtain a special waiver. Research teams should prepare for such factors well in advance. We are far away from a universal stance on this issue, and any approach taken will need to consider the research and the context, as such, and researchers like the ones who wrote this case are advised to keep sharing the perspectives of their participants who find such requirements alienating.

Case 7.3 Responding to concerns about participant burden and vulnerability in health-related action research in Ireland

Geralyn Hynes

Introduction

This case is written by an academic working in palliative care in Ireland, whose plans to undertake action research with patients with advanced chronic respiratory disease were thwarted by research ethics committees. Irish policy recognises three levels of palliative care expertise: specialist, intermediate and basic. For the basic level, everyone with direct involvement in patient care must have basic palliative care skills and competencies. Despite widespread support across the Irish health service for the policy, there are persistent problems in embedding basic level palliative care across the system.

The case

I was interested to know how basic level palliative care might be embedded in everyday nursing care and in so doing, to: 1) better understand the general problem with implementing this policy; 2) seek ways of addressing the palliative care needs of patients with advanced chronic respiratory disease – as these patients experience a heavy symptom burden and frequent admissions to hospital. I decided on an action research approach as this had potential to provide insights into why a policy that is so well-supported should prove so difficult to implement. I focused on nursing practice following an approach by a respiratory nurse specialist to support her efforts to address palliative care needs of her patients.

I understood palliative care as being philosophically different to what I saw as the standard disease-oriented approach to care of patients in our acute hospitals. Palliative care draws attention to the interdependence of physical, psychosocial, emotional, and spiritual or existential dimensions of advanced illness experience. The more standard disease-oriented approach to care reflects a biomedical reductionist stance to understanding and managing symptoms.

I formed a planning group involving interested respiratory nurses from the participating hospital and introduced the idea of action research. The nurses had not previously experienced action research but expressed strong support for it. My engagement was guided by my understanding of action research specifically, co-operative inquiry.

Ultimately, we arrived at a proposal to establish an action research group that would be comprised of nurses and patients and would:

1. guide my information gathering on and analysis of palliative care needs of the patient cohort;
2. guide the development and implementation of palliative care strategies across the hospital.

In keeping with local requirements, we applied to two separate research ethics committees namely, the University's Faculty Research Ethics Committee and the Hospital's Research Ethics Committee. Both involve separate processes and application forms. The proposal was rejected by the Faculty Research Ethics Committee on the grounds that a) including patients who had advanced disease in an action research group would be too onerous for them, and b) asking patients to engage in a project the outcome of which was not pre-determined in terms of activities and time was unacceptable. The rejection meant that the application to the Hospital's Research Ethics Committee had to be withdrawn.

For the planning group, the rejection meant returning to the drawing board to develop a new proposal. We were clear that patients should be involved because of their experiences of symptom burden and care across different services within the hospital. However, the nurses viewed the rejection as symptomatic of the dominant narratives of a medical hierarchical system and institutional practices.

The nurses believed that in order to get support for changes in practice, we needed to produce data using well-recognised measures to assess care needs. This troubled me because it went against the tenets of action research that were guiding my collaboration with the nurses and project as a whole, namely that participation in action research is both epistemological and political. In other words, the nature and quality of participation determines the kind of knowledge produced. Using well-recognised instruments with closed questions was, to me, denying patient participants the scope to tell their stories and explore how the hospital might attend to these through palliative care. I understood the nurses' concerns but was acutely aware that we were making decisions about the project design before they had a strong feel for action research, and the implications for knowledge production.

Ultimately, a new two-phased proposal was developed. Phase one proposed structured interviews with patients in their own homes using well-recognised disease-specific health status measures. Phase two proposed a cooperative inquiry group comprised of interested nurses. Though interested patients would be invited to attend up to three cooperative inquiry meetings to provide commentary and ideas, they would not be actively engaged in the action research. The proposal was approved by both ethics committees.

However, when interviewed, patient participants treated the closed questions as discussion points. After a pilot interview, I decided to record and capture the stories that were prompted by the questions allowing discussion and follow-up questions to flow. I successfully sought an amendment to my application to both committees to allow this approach. Phase one findings ultimately provided rich ground for exploring not just the patients' unmet palliative care needs but also, their suggestions as to how needs might be best addressed.

On the face of it, failure to get ethics approval for the initial proposal meant there was limited scope for patients to meaningfully engage with the nurses on how care-practices and the service as a whole could be developed. Our second application ran the risk of producing findings that would simply confirm what we already knew about unmet palliative care needs, rather than producing practical knowledge about how these needs can be addressed within the system. By interrogating how I, as a researcher, can consciously attend to participation and how knowledge is produced, I was able to give greater ownership of the interview process to patients. This approach went beyond simply hearing their stories; it allowed conversations about palliative care needs to unfold. These stories and conversations formed the basis for the work of the cooperative inquiry group. Ultimately, the project produced actions to target suffering which reflected palliative care.

Hospital Ethics Committees are more familiar with dealing with highly structured and predictable research trajectories than the unfolding process and principles that characterise action research. Hospital-based action research projects are typically collaborative involving staff with little or no action research experience. The researcher's own immersion in action research principles and ways of being will ultimately influence the degree to which these early challenges are met.

Commentary on Case 7.3

Adrian Guta

This case highlights a frustrating situation in which an ethical review board made paternalistic assumptions about participants at the end of life. It is very disappointing to hear that such a proposal was 'rejected' and without much constructive feedback from the board. Persons at the end of life are indeed a vulnerable group and may be highly dependent on their health care providers, but this needs to be balanced with their desire to inform future research and care. The requirement to have predetermined activities and times for an action research group, which is very different than a participant in a regular project, shows a lack of understanding on the part of the ethical review committee. In my work with persons experiencing advanced illness residing in a hospital, they have been very open about their limitations (e.g., 'I am unable to attend long research team meetings because of my health') and letting the team know when they need to leave the project to focus on personal and health matters. It is disappointing that this ethical review board only saw them as passive. In this case the researcher accepted the decision but insisted on honouring the narratives of participants and going back to the ethical review board with an amendment. This had a positive ending, but it might not have gone this way with another board. Regardless, the researcher made an informed decision to meet the needs of participants at the moment. Participatory researchers may regularly encounter participants who want to deviate from the researcher's script or protocol. These need to be considered on a case by case basis, but it is helpful to integrate this into future ethical review submissions as evidence.

Case 7.4 Dilemmas in a UK PAR project involving mental health service users and providers

Jon Fieldhouse

Introduction

This case was contributed by a community mental health assertive outreach (AO) practitioner in the UK. AO services aim to meet the needs of people with severe mental health challenges who do not wish to use services or have difficulty doing so. This work focuses on recovery and social inclusion; addressing needs related to accommodation, occupational deprivation, drug or alcohol addiction, self-neglect, and possible challenging behaviour.

The case

Following the UK government's Social Exclusion Unit's report, I was seconded to lead a Bristol-wide project implementing the national social inclusion agenda. This promoted service users' re-integration into the mainstream community via voluntary work, education, training, or employment, for example.

As a practitioner, I saw that much learning could potentially be derived from the experiences of AO service users; many of whom had become well-engaged with mainstream community activities despite the received wisdom (amongst service providers) that they would not achieve this without segregated day hospital support. In practice, the 'AO service user experience' contested these work-cultural assumptions and I felt spurred to explore this conundrum. I secured funds from the National Institute of Mental Health in England to initiate a PAR process. I wanted to interview the AO service users and use that learning to inform the work of a roundtable group of mental health and non-mental health professionals and mental health service users who were focused on improving service users' access to the kind of mainstream life opportunities noted earlier. I anticipated that the AO service users themselves would be able to join the group to represent their own experience. However, while the PAR did help joint-working by professionals across health and social care sectors – with one group member saying it felt 'as if a wall was being dismantled from both sides' – the inclusion of AO service users proved harder to facilitate.

As a practitioner member of the working group and principal investigator for the PAR, the first ethical dilemma I faced was when the ethics committee regarded AO service users' vulnerability as a basis for precluding their membership of the working group. Ethical concerns revolved around *informed consent* about the research process, participants' *rights to privacy* (given that participation would involve self-disclosure as local service users), and *protection from harm* (such as anxiety or emotional distress).

Any research involving NHS patients (or their data) in England must be approved by the Health Research Authority (HRA), a subsidiary body of the Department of Health. HRA approval combines assessment of research governance and legal compliance and scrutiny by a research ethics committee to ensure research activities uphold participants' dignity, rights, safety and well-being.

Following the ethics board decision, I had to find a way to ensure adequate follow-through from the interviews into the working group because there was now an alarming discontinuity between the service users who provided interview data and those who might subsequently act on the learning in the working group. I felt that central tenets of PAR – its widened epistemology and its democracy, for example – were being compromised.

I wondered about feeding the interview findings into the working group as dis-embodied 'data', but this seemed more like research *for* people than *with* them. If direct experiential knowing about what had 'worked' was so valuable, by what right was it to be 'taken away' from an already marginalised group? I also wondered whether participation through qualitative interviews was still 'participation' in PAR terms, or a kind of *pseudo*-participation?

I decided to improvise, on the basis of a firm ethical commitment to the credibility of the qualitative data. Even if the AO interviewees took no further part in the PAR, their uniquely valuable data was a rare ingredient in NHS research which might yet help us understand how (so-called) 'difficult to engage' people had become so well-engaged.

To this end, I invited two service user researchers from Bristol MIND (a mental health charity) and two additional service users to join the PAR steering group. Although the service user members had not been interviewees, one was a sibling of an AO service user who understood the importance of accessing an authentic AO service user voice in research. Furthermore, the likely power imbalance of having an AO practitioner (myself) as an interviewer was mitigated by involvement of MIND service user researchers as co-designers of the interview schedule, as co-interviewers, and as data co-analysts. This greatly helped the credibility and impact of the interview findings when disseminated.

As the PAR unfolded over its 20-month lifespan, the transmission of momentum was nevertheless problematic. Because the AO service users' experience of by-passing the need for day services ran contrary to the accepted organisational narrative, it was doubted by senior decision-makers. This impasse prompted me to engage the late Dr. Sue Porter, an external PAR facilitator from the Centre for Action Research in Professional Practice (CAARP), to lead two co-operative inquiry workshops. This 'outsider' perspective highlighted the need for the inclusion of more senior managers in dialogue, and significantly shifted the PAR's focus towards examining how organisational systems learn and innovate. This created some anxiety amongst PAR participants about potential conflict with managers who commissioned the services they worked in or used, raising ethical questions about confidentiality, anonymity, informed consent and the avoidance of harm.

The social exclusion and stigmatisation of mental health service users means they have a special claim for protection from harm and assured confidentiality during research. Yet, balanced against this is PAR's drive to improve people's lives and engage the voices of *all* stakeholders in knowledge creation, particularly service users' voices. Learning about this tension between PAR's *principles* and its *methods* (where adapting design in the thick of the action may increase participants' exposure to stressors and/or loss of confidentiality) has made me more aware of the friction this creates with traditional deontological ethical scrutiny, with its one-off, predictive 'snapshot' approach.

Commentary on Case 7.4

Adrian Guta

This case highlights the discontinuity between the concerns identified by the ethical review committee and those which arose in the field. It is disappointing to hear that a review committee deemed participants unable to join a working group based on paternalistic notions of informed consent, privacy, and potential emotional risks. The consumer survivor literature includes strong arguments about the importance of involving persons with lived experience of mental illness in decision-making and many mental health institutions involve service users in programme development. The case further illustrates how the decisions from the ethical review board necessitated a series of ongoing decisions to fill an important gap which ultimately may have brought in expert external stakeholders that undermined the trust of participants. Participatory researchers are often required to make ongoing decisions during the life of projects and may not be comfortable approaching their ethical review board for advice. In my own research with participatory researchers many expressed that they are working with a trial and error approach because they do not feel they can approach their ethical review boards for guidance.

PART 3: CONCLUDING COMMENTS

This chapter has explored tensions which may emerge when participatory researchers encounter ethical review boards and requirements which assume a traditional positivistic research design with clear separation between the researcher and researched. Traditional review models have universal elements which should be considered by all researchers, but may not be suited to the kinds of relationships and approaches found in participatory research. My goal has been to emphasise the potential of working with ethical review boards in a productive way which grounds the ethical review submission in community norms and related scholarship to assure boards of the legitimacy of participatory research and using alternative approaches for ensuring participant protections. Several of the cases included in this chapter highlight ways in which researchers challenged their ethical review boards and were able to proceed in desired ways. Other cases highlight a lack of responsiveness from ethical review boards which resulted in researchers being put in uncomfortable situations and potentially compromised the experience of participants. When ethical review boards lack knowledge about participatory research approaches they may be overly protectionist and paternalistic while simultaneously missing important opportunities to prepare researchers for the complexities of the work they are undertaking. In closing, I wish to reemphasise the tremendous learning that I acquired by having both roles. I strongly recommend that participatory researchers join their ethical review committees and bring their knowledge to the table, as well as sharing it in important forums like this book.

References

Allen, G. (2008). Getting Beyond Form Filling: The Role of Institutional Governance in Human Research Ethics. *Journal of Academic Ethics, 6*(2), 105–116. doi:10.1007/s10805-008-9057-9

Ashcroft, R. E. (1999). The new national statement on ethical conduct in research involving humans: A social theoretic perspective. *Monash Bioethics Review, 18*(4-Ethics Committee Supplement), 14–17.

Ashcroft, R. E., & Pfeffer, N. (2001). Ethics behind closed doors: Do research ethics committees need secrecy? *British Medical Journal, 322*(7297), 1294–1296.

Babbie, E. (2004). Laud Humphreys and research ethics. *International Journal of Sociology and Social Policy, 24*(3/4/5), 12–19.

Banks, S., Armstrong, A., Carter, K., Graham, H., Hayward, P., Henry, A., . . . Strachan, A. (2013). Everyday ethics in community-based participatory research. *Contemporary Social Science, 8*(3), 263–277. doi:10.1080/21582041.2013.769618

Bean, S., & Silva, D. S. (2010). Betwixt & Between: Peer Recruiter Proximity in Community-Based Research. *The American Journal of Bioethics, 10*(3), 18–19. doi:10.1080/15265160903581783

Blake, M. K. (2007). Formality and friendship: research ethics review and participatory action research. *ACME, 6*(3), 411–421.

Boser, S. (2006). Ethics and power in community-campus partnerships for research. *Action Research, 4*(1), 9–21.

Boser, S. (2007). Power, ethics, and the IRB: Dissonance over human participant review of participatory research. *Qualitative Inquiry, 13*(8), 1060–1074.

Chabot, C., Shoveller, J. A., Spencer, G., & Johnson, J. L. (2012). Ethical and Epistemological Insights: A Case Study of Participatory Action Research with Young People. *Journal of Empirical Research on Human Research Ethics, 7*(2), 20–33. doi:10.1525/jer.2012.7.2.20

Chadwick, G. L. (1997). Historical perspective: Nuremberg, Tuskegee, and the radiation experiments. *J Int Assoc Physicians AIDS Care, 3*(1), 27–28.

Coleman, C., & Bouesseau, M.-C. (2008). How do we know that research ethics committees are really working? The neglected role of outcomes assessment in research ethics review. *BMC Medical Ethics, 9*(1), 6.

Constantine, M. (2010). Disentangling Methodologies: The Ethics of Traditional Sampling Methodologies, Community-Based Participatory Research, and Respondent-Driven Sampling. *The American Journal of Bioethics, 10*(3), 22–24. doi:10.1080/15265160903585628

Dingwall, R. (2008). The ethical case against ethical regulation in humanities and social science research. *Contemporary Social Science: Journal of the Academy of Social Sciences, 3*(1), 1–12.

Downie, J., & Cottrell, B. (2001). Community-based research ethics review: Reflections on experience and recommendations for action. *Health law review, 10*(1), 8–17.

Fitzpatrick, E. F., Martiniuk, A. L., D'Antoine, H., Oscar, J., Carter, M., & Elliott, E. J. (2016). Seeking consent for research with indigenous communities: A systematic review. *BMC Medical Ethics, 17*(1), 65.

Flicker, S., & Guta, A. (2008). Ethical approaches to adolescent participation in sexual health research. *Journal of Adolescent Health, 42*(1), 3–10.

Flicker, S., Guta, A., Larkin, J., Flynn, S., Fridkin, A., Pole, J., . . . Chan., K. (2010). Survey Design From the Ground Up: Collaboratively Creating the Toronto Teen Survey. *Health Promotion Practice, 11*(1), 112–122.

Flicker, S., O'Campo, P., Monchalin, R., Thistle, J., Worthington, C., Masching, R., ... Thomas, C. (2015). Research done in "a good way": The importance of Indigenous elder involvement in HIV community-based research. *American Journal of Public Health, 105*(6), 1149–1154.

Flicker, S., Roche, B., & Guta, A. (2010). *Peer research in action III: Ethical issues.* Toronto: Wellesley Institute.

Flicker, S., Travers, R., Guta, A., McDonald, S., & Meagher, A. (2007). Ethical Dilemmas in Community-Based Participatory Research: Recommendations for Institutional Review Boards. *Journal of Urban Health, 84*(4), 478–493. doi:10.1007/s11524-007-9165-7

Freimuth, V. S., Quinn, S. C., Thomas, S. B., Cole, G., Zook, E., & Duncan, T. (2001). African Americans' views on research and the Tuskegee Syphilis Study. *Social Science & Medicine, 52*(5), 797–808.

Green, L. A., Lowery, J. C., Kowalski, C. P., & Wyszewianski, L. (2006). Impact of Institutional Review Board Practice Variation on Observational Health Services Research. *Health Services Research, 41*(1), 214–230. doi:10.1111/j.1475-6773.2005.00458.x

Greene, S., Ahluwalia, A., Watson, J., Tucker, R., Rourke, S. B., Koornstra, J., . . . Byers, S. (2009). Between skepticism and empowerment: the experiences of peer research assistants in HIV/AIDS, housing and homelessness community-based research. *International Journal of Social Research Methodology, 12*(4), 361–373.

Grodin, M. A., & Annas, G. J. (1996). Legacies of Nuremberg: Medical ethics and human rights. *JAMA, 276*(20), 1682–1683.

Guillemin, M., & Gillam, L. (2004). Ethics, Reflexivity, and "Ethically Important Moments" in Research. *Qualitative Inquiry, 10*(2), 261–280. doi:10.1177/1077800403262360

Guta, A., Flicker, S., & Roche, B. (2010). *Peer research in action II: Management, support and supervision.* Toronto: Wellesley Institute.

Guta, A., Flicker, S., & Roche, B. (2013). Governing through community allegiance: A qualitative examination of peer research in community-based participatory research. *Critical public health, 23*(4), 432–451.

Guta, A., Murray, S. J., Strike, C., Flicker, S., Upshur, R., & Myers, T. (2016). Governing Well in Community-Based Research: Lessons from Canada's HIV Research Sector on Ethics, Publics and the Care of the Self. *Public Health Ethics*, 10(3), 315–328. doi. org/10.1093/phe/phw024.

Guta, A., Nixon, S., Gahagan, J., & Fielden, S. (2012). "Walking along beside the researcher": How Canadian REBs/IRBs are responding to the needs of community-based participatory research. *Journal of Empirical Research on Human Research Ethics, 7*(1), 17–27.

Guta, A., Nixon, S. A., & Wilson, M. G. (2013). Resisting the seduction of "ethics creep": Using Foucault to surface complexity and contradiction in research ethics review. *Social Science & Medicine, 98*, 301–310. doi.org/10.1016/j.socscimed.2012.09.019.

Guta, A., Wilson, M. G., Flicker, S., Travers, R., Mason, C., Wenyeve, G., & O'Campo, P. (2010). Are we asking the right questions? A review of Canadian REB practices in relation to community-based participatory research. *Journal of Empirical Research on Human Research Ethics, 5*(2), 35–46.

Haggerty, K. D. (2004). Ethics Creep: Governing Social Science Research in the Name of Ethics. *Qualitative Sociology, 27*(4), 391–414.

Hoeyer, K. (2006). "Ethics wars": Reflections on the Antagonism between Bioethicists and Social Science Observers of Biomedicine. *Human Studies, 29*(2), 203–227.

Hoeyer, K., Dahlager, L., & Lynoe, N. (2005). Conflicting notions of research ethics. The mutually challenging traditions of social scientists and medical researchers. *Social Science & Medicine, 61*(8), 1741–1749. doi:S0277-9536(05)00121-8 [pii]10.1016/j. socscimed.2005.03.026

Horowitz, C. R., Robinson, M., & Seifer, S. (2009). Community-based participatory research from the margin to the mainstream. *Circulation, 119*(19), 2633–2642.

Humphreys, L. (1970). *Tearoom trade: Impersonal sex in public places.* Chicago: Aldine Pub. Co.

International Compilation of Human Research Protections. (2017). International Compilation of Human Research Protections. Retrieved from http://www.hhs.gov/ohrp/international/intlcompilation/intlcompilation.html (accessed January 2018).

Jones, J. H. (1993). *Bad blood: The Tuskegee syphilis experiment* (New and expanded ed.). Toronto: Maxwell Macmillan Canada.

Jürgens, R. (2005). *"Nothing about us without us"–greater, meaningful involvement of people who use illegal drugs: a public health, ethical, and human rights imperative*: Canadian HIV/AIDS Legal Network.

Krugman, S. (1986). The Willowbrook hepatitis studies revisited: Ethical aspects. *Reviews of Infectious Diseases, 8*(1), 157–162.

Lewis, M. (2008). New Strategies of Control: Academic Freedom and Research Ethics Boards. *Qualitative Inquiry, 14*(5), 684–699. doi:10.1177/1077800408314347

Logie, C., James, L., Tharao, W., & Loutfy, M. R. (2012). Opportunities, ethical challenges, and lessons learned from working with peer research assistants in a multi-method HIV community-based research study in Ontario, Canada. *Journal of Empirical Research on Human Research Ethics, 7*(4), 10–19.

Marshall, Z., Nixon, S., Nepveux, D., Vo, T., Wilson, C., Flicker, S., . . . Proudfoot, D. (2012). Navigating risks and professional roles: Research with lesbian, gay, bisexual, trans, and queer young people with intellectual disabilities. *Journal of Empirical Research on Human Research Ethics, 7*(4), 20–33.

Martin, D. (2007). Bureacratizing ethics: Institutional review boards and participatory research. *ACME, 6*(3), 319–328.

Milgram, S. (1974). *Obedience to authority:An experimental view* (1st ed.). New York: Harper & Row.

Morgan, M. F., Cuskelly, M., & Moni, K. B. (2014). Unanticipated ethical issues in a participatory research project with individuals with intellectual disability. *Disability & Society, 29*(8), 1305–-1318.

O'Reilly, M., Dixon-Woods, M., Angell, E., Ashcroft, R. E., & Bryman, A. (2009). Doing accountability: A discourse analysis of research ethics committee letters. *Sociol Health Illness, 31*(2), 246–261.

Office of the Secretary. (1979). *The Belmont Report: Ethical Principles and Guidelines for the Protection of Human Subjects of Research last retrieved on Nov 15, 2005 from http://www.hhs.gov/ohrp/humansubjects/guidance/belmont.htm*. Retrieved from Washington, DC:

Reverby, S. (2009). *Examining Tuskegee: The infamous syphilis study and its legacy*. Chapel Hill: University of North Carolina Press.

Roche, B., Flicker, S., & Guta, A. (2010). *Peer research in action I: Models of practice*. Toronto: Wellesley Institute.

Rolfe, G. (2005). Colliding discourses: Deconstructing the process of seeking ethical approval for a participatory evaluation project. *NT Research, 10*(2), 231–231.

Rothman, D. J. (1982). Were Tuskegee & Willowbrook 'studies in nature'? *Hastings Cent Rep, 12*(2), 5–7.

Savulescu, J., Chalmers, I., & Blunt, J. (1996). Are research ethics committees behaving unethically? Some suggestions for improving performance and accountability. *BMJ, 313*(7069), 1390–1393.

Shore, N. (2006). Re-Conceptualizing the Belmont Report: A Community-Based Participatory Research Perspective. *Journal of Community Practice, 14*(4), 5–26.

Simon, C., & Mosavel, M. (2010). Community Members as Recruiters of Human Subjects: Ethical Considerations. *The American Journal of Bioethics, 10*(3), 3–11. doi:10.1080/15265160903585578

Solomon, S., & Piechowski, P. J. (2011). Developing Community Partner Training: Regulations and Relationships. *Journal of Empirical Research on Human Research Ethics, 6*(2), 23–30. doi:10.1525/jer.2011.6.2.23

Strike, C., Guta, A., De Prinse, K., Switzer, S., & Carusone, S. C. (2016). Opportunities, challenges and ethical issues associated with conducting community-based participatory research in a hospital setting. *Research Ethics, 12*(3), 149–157.

Switzer, S., Guta, A., de Prinse, K., Carusone, S. C., & Strike, C. (2015). Visualizing harm reduction: Methodological and ethical considerations. *Social Science & Medicine, 133,* 77–84.

The Nuremberg Code. (1949). "Permissible Medical Experiments." Trials of War Criminals before the Nuremberg Military Tribunals under Control Council Law No. 10. Nuremberg October 1946 – April 1949, Washington. U.S. Government Printing Office (n.d.), vol. 2., pp. 181–182. REPRINTED in 1996. *Journal of the American Medical Association, 276*(20), 1691.

Upshur, R. E. G. (2011). Ask not what your REB can do for you; ask what you can do for your REB. *Canadian Family Physician, 57*(10), 1113–1114.

Wolf, L. E. (2010). The research ethics committee is not the enemy: Oversight of community-based participatory research. *Journal of Empirical Research on Human Research Ethics, 5*(4), 77–86.

World Medical Association Declaration of Helsinki. (1964). Ethical principles for medical research involving human subjects (last amended Oct 2000). Retrieved November 15, 2005, from www.wma.net/e/policy/b3.htm.

Zimbardo, P. G. (1973). On the ethics of intervention in human psychological research: With special reference to the Stanford Prison Experiment. *Cognition, 2*(2), 243–256.

8

SOCIAL ACTION FOR SOCIAL CHANGE

Erin Davis and Cathy Vaughan

With cases contributed by Saskia Duijs, Vivianne Baur, Raquel Ignacio, Philile Mbatha and Jasmin Chen

PART 1: INTRODUCTION AND OVERVIEW

Erin Davis and Cathy Vaughan

Background

This chapter introduction is written from our perspectives as community-based researchers using participatory approaches in various settings in Australia and elsewhere. Erin locates herself as a white Canadian-Australian woman and migrant living on the unceded territories of the Kulin Nation in Melbourne. Her background combines critical social work, community-based participatory research and policy advocacy primarily on issues related to gender equality and violence against women. Erin has recently completed a Master's thesis focusing on the ethics of action and social change in participatory research. Cathy is a white, middle-class, public health practitioner who does not have lived experience of disability. She has a PhD in social psychology, and has worked with non-government organisations in various settings in Australia, Asia and the Pacific. She is now university-based, working primarily with immigrant and refugee women, women with disabilities, and community-based organisations to conduct research on reducing health inequalities.

We believe that reflexivity about our social location is a critical aspect of ethical participatory research and important for understanding how our own experiences and backgrounds inform our ideas about what constitutes effective action. Awareness of our social position is essential when working in community settings with people who are often marginalised by social inequality and structural oppression, and do not have the same access as we do to social privilege, institutional power and resources. This also makes us aware that contributing to social change through participatory research requires undertaking forms of action relevant within community contexts, beyond traditional academic outputs. There is limited guidance in the participatory research field, however, on how action and social change should be conceptualised and ethically enacted.

To address this, we begin in Part 1 by exploring the theoretical underpinnings and conceputalisations of action and social change in participatory research. This is followed by considering the impacts of power on progressing change outcomes and finishes with discussion about an ethical framework of reflexivity and solidarity to guide researchers and community members in maximising possibilities for action and contribution to social change.

In Part 2, we use this reflexive-solidarity framework to comment on four cases contributed by researchers grappling with ethical issues encountered in working for social change in different global settings. Case 8.1 explores the complexities of tackling action and social change in research involving multicultural women in a disenfranchised neighbourhood in the Netherlands. Case 8.2 critiques how participatory research 'shakes up' the status quo for women with disabilities in the Philippines, compelling their interest in taking further action on their reproductive health rights, but without sustainable resources to do so. In Case 8.3, research in South Africa reminds us of the importance of understanding local community power dynamics and historical contexts to support grassroots action and build social change movements. Lastly, Case 8.4 presents tensions arising when researchers and community members have differing values and perspectives about how action and social change are understood when confronting violence against women in Australia.

In Part 3, we return to the importance of dialogically engaging with community members, other allies and stakeholders about desired action to transform research outcomes into meaningful contributions to social justice.

Theoretical foundations of action in participatory research

The emergence of participatory research signified an ontological turn from the traditional conventions of empirical positivism toward a 'participatory worldview' by combining critical theory (such as Marxism, feminism and post-colonialism) with 'constructivism', recognising that knowledge is produced through an interaction of complex social, cultural and historical realities that researchers and participants alike bring to the research engagement. In a participatory worldview, knowledge is transformed into action to address social disadvantage and progress social change and emancipatory outcomes (Reason & Bradbury, 2006). Researchers seeking to apply this participatory worldview often draw on Paulo Freire's (1970) notion of 'praxis', that is, action based on 'critical consciousness': the tipping point where people gain awareness and knowledge about the impacts of structural oppression on their lives, compelling them to take action against systems that perpetuate domination and inequality.

These theoretical foundations motivate researchers to use participatory, rather than 'traditional', approaches both in recognition of the expertise and rights of

community members and from a desire to directly address disadvantage and contribute to social change (Wallerstein & Duran, 2008). To ignore the social change
goals of participatory research not only undermines its potential, but also denies
justice to the very people who give so much of themselves in the research process
as they expose their inner worlds, challenges and suffering sometimes in the face
of personal risk.

Conceptualising action and social change

Guidance on the 'participatory' aspects of participatory research typically out-
lines approaches to engaging researchers and community members in a range of
research design processes such as defining the research problem; creating research
questions; choosing and implementing methods for data collection and analysis;
and designing formats and tactics for dissemination of results (Castleden et al.,
2012). There has been less consideration, however, of what exactly constitutes
the 'action' component of this research approach and how action in participatory
research might contribute to 'social change' (Reid et al., 2006). Furthermore,
descriptions of community members' own conceptualisations of action are scarce.
This leaves researchers with limited guidance to transform the knowledge and
capacities constructed through the research engagement into tangible outcomes.
Participatory researchers are often left wondering if their efforts will make a difference in the lives of community members and address issues of disadvantage at
a broader level.

While specific guidelines and investigations into action and social change in
participatory research are limited, we have found that descriptions of these concepts in the relevant literature can generally be categorised as three different, but
interrelated, forms:

1) transformative individual or group level change;
2) social action arising from individual and group level change; and
3) broader social change at systemic and structural levels.

Individual and group level change (1) can emerge through the 'participatory'
practices that involve co-constructing knowledge and developing practical skills,
leading to increased psychosocial resources and new collaborative connections
(Vaughan et al., 2014; George et al., 2007; Foster-Fishman et al., 2005). These
changes may enable critical consciousness, as individuals and groups take social
action (2) to improve their own health and well-being, and possibly also the health
and well-being of others in their communities. Participatory researchers describe
the busy eruptions of social action that arise during and as a result of research projects, often through short-term activities on the part of community members and
collaborators (Vaughan, 2014; Nygreen, 2009; Reid et al., 2006). As George et al.
(2007) suggest, 'participatory research can provide opportunities by which people
gain skills and a sense of the possibilities for social change', that support 'actions by

which people, individually and collectively, take control of their environment' (p. 182).

When social action does emerge from the praxis of participatory research, this in turn may contribute to broader social change (point 3 above). By social change, we mean larger-scale changes and socio-political alterations that contribute to the redistribution of power and resources through changes to policy, legislation, systems, and social relationships and structures. As such, while individual and group level change is important and positive, the transformative potential of participatory research needs to be of sustainable benefit to the wider community in order to contribute to social change. Case 8.3 offers insights into this as the author describes how a research project both enabled and intertwined with social change activities taken up by community members who were resisting power-over dynamics from village authorities as part of their efforts to gain more control over their lives. Increased knowledge about their rights gained through participation in the research project gave rise to further opportunities for community members to contribute to decision-making platforms about policies that impact the wider community.

Importantly, this shift from individual to collective impact cannot be assumed. For example, in documenting the positive impact of a participatory research project in depressed areas of Michigan, Foster-Fishman et al. (2005) note that their project was a catalyst for action in a context where there was political will and resources available for neighbourhood improvement. They question whether the project could in fact have been disempowering if the participatory research process had increased awareness of the need for change in the absence of opportunities and political support for local people to actually take tangible action. Cornish (2006) also observes that the potential psychosocial benefits of participation, such as self-confidence and a sense of alternative futures, are valuable resources to community members involved in participatory research; however, genuine empowerment involves participants gaining concrete structural power to make changes in their material circumstances. Cornish and others question whether disadvantaged community members themselves should be entirely responsible for the actions necessary to bring about social change. Similarly, Ledwith (2007) argues that the potential for social change is hindered by a focus on the 'immediate, local and specific', which may confine actions emerging from research to addressing the symptoms of social disparity rather than tackling the root causes of structural oppression (p. 597).

Chatterton, Fuller and Routledge (2007) suggest that one pathway from individual/group level change to broader social change at systemic and structural levels, is through advocating to those in power, arguing that 'our encounters are therefore not just about action in the research process, but how the research process can contribute to wider activism such as protests, demonstrations, events and campaigns to effect change' (p. 221). Participatory researchers can learn from social movements and how these contribute to change, by both building the skills and confidence of disadvantaged groups and investing in actions that motivate power-brokers to attend to the 'push from below' (Campbell et al., 2010). Community advocates describe how they value researchers' efforts 'to help us voice our concerns effectively, tap into resources for community improvement, and challenge the status quo, as necessary, to achieve community goals' (Van der Eb et al., 2004, p. 222).

It is difficult, however, to see a linear relationship between actions in participatory research and sustainable social change outcomes. We must acknowledge that social change is generated by the persistent efforts of individuals and collectives taking a multitude of actions in diverse contexts. Participatory research is just one contributor alongside activist campaigning, political reform, legislative change and other movements seeking to redress inequality. For example, our experience conducting participatory research with immigrant and refugee women about their experiences of domestic violence is situated within current and historical social change efforts working to prevent and redress the harms of violence against women and also advance the rights and status of migrants and refugees. We are acutely aware that the impact of our research findings would be very limited if we did not link them with the existing advocacy efforts of community partners. This has allowed our research findings to be utilised in current domestic violence systemic reforms, contribute to professional and community education programmes, and create new community resources that centralise immigrant and refugee women's voices.

The impact of power on action and change

It is necessary to recognise that these three interrelated forms of action and social change are almost always shaped by differential access to resources, social inequalities, cultural norms, political contexts and historical relationships. Although participatory research is premised on egalitarian ideals, it is not immune to the operations of power at relational and systemic levels (Banks et al., 2013; Golob & Giles, 2013; Castleden et al., 2012).

Institutional power

An obvious power differential that shapes action outcomes in participatory research involves those who are institutionally employed researchers (i.e. within universities, community organisations, government departments) and the community members who live with the disadvantages relevant to the social and health issues being examined. These differences are often reinforced by the power of the institutions that typically control participatory research projects. Unchecked institutional control can conflict with the democratic principles upon which participatory research is based, and may reproduce the dominating power dynamics seen in conventional research (Golob & Giles, 2013). This is highly problematic when participatory research methods are used, intentionally or otherwise, to co-opt people into projects that end up positioning them as responsible for overcoming the conditions in which they experience disadvantage, rather than directing action against the structures and systems that make such disadvantage possible in the first place (Jordan & Kapoor, 2016). This may be particularly evident where actions arising from participatory research are situated only at the individual/group level and power imbalances block the shift to sustained social change.

Institutional power and control can also constrain action by placing unrealistic limitations on research timelines and funding resources. A lack of funding and adequate time to allow participatory research relationships to grow and flourish can reinforce the view that institutions are not genuinely committed to seeing research through to the point of supporting social change outcomes. It can also leave community members with the challenge of sustaining the momentum required to pursue action emerging from the original research engagement (Caldwell, et al., 2015; Van der Eb, et al., 2004). This is illustrated in Case 8.2, where women with disabilities in the Philippines struggled to continue activities originally supported by research funding.

This critique of institutional power does not mean that universities and other research-focused institutions are disinterested in progressing positive change outcomes. In recent years there has been a growing international focus on the 'impact' of research. Research funders in many countries are increasingly requiring demonstrations of impact by showing a direct relationship between research investment and social and economic change; however, the impact agenda presents specific challenges for researchers who prioritise working with the social action efforts of local communities for more radical social justice purposes (Banks et al., 2017; Darby, 2017). Participatory researchers have highlighted that frameworks for measuring, and assigning value to, research impact tend to prioritise scale and reach (Evans, 2016), privileging certain forms and sources of evidence over community perspectives (Fine, 2012). Measurement of impact favours forms of evidence that are based on the assumption that change occurring as a result of academic research is linear, occurs at the completion of a project, and is predictable and quantifiable (Banks et al., 2017; Darby, 2017; Evans, 2016). This is in contrast to participatory researchers' experience of research contributions to social change as dynamic, unpredictable, qualitative and relational.

Power dynamics within communities

It is also necessary to recognise that action and change are influenced by power dynamics at the community level. As Yoshihama and Carr (2002) note: 'communities are not places that researchers enter but are instead a set of negotiations that inherently entail multiple and often conflicting interests' (p. 99). Depending on the sensitivities of the research subject and the power dynamics at play, some people may be in a position to participate while others may be excluded (Minkler, 2004), For example, the social actions emergent from participatory research may only represent the interests of those individuals who become involved in research projects, or who hold powerful community gatekeeping roles (Banks, et al., 2013). This is illustrated in Case 8.3, when initially it was the 'headmen' in a rural area of South Africa who authorised the research project on behalf of hesitant community members.

When only a few people are called upon to represent a community and speak to social and health issues that have community-wide impact, the knowledge that is produced may not be accepted by others who are affected by research outcomes. Individual and group based social actions may then be challenged in this context. Additionally, some people may be restricted from full participation because of the burdens of intensive involvement in participatory research, and barriers caused by the very disadvantages the research seeks to understand.

Researchers must also operate carefully in community settings and broader socio-political climates that may be hostile to challenges to entrenched power structures both within communities and at broader levels (Minkler, 2004). While taking action with aims toward social change is idealised, in reality it can also create problems for those who have the most to lose if their activities are met with indifference or antagonism (Reid, et al., 2006).

An ethical framework of reflexivity and solidarity

We recognise that there is considerable overlap between the three interrelated forms of action and change, and understand that the operations of power in participatory research are complicated, contextual and dynamic. This very complexity highlights the ethical imperative on the part of those who undertake participatory research to consider how the concepts of action and social change might be understood and applied. Without in-depth consideration of these concepts, there is a risk of disappointment, unmet expectations, disempowerment and disagreement over the purpose of engaging in participatory research and determining the potential reach of its outcomes. It is not simply a matter of following through on the promise of a participatory approach, but of working ethically with people who participate in research and hold justified expectations that their participation will somehow alleviate disadvantage. What then are the ethics that researchers can utilise to maximise the possibilities for social action toward social change, while also addressing the operations of power that commonly constrain action in participatory research endeavours? We suggest a framework based in the ethics of reflexivity and solidarity.

The centrality of reflexivity

In qualitative research, reflexivity is described as 'the ability to reflect inward toward oneself as an inquirer; outward to the cultural, historical, linguistic, political, and other forces that shape everything about inquiry; and, in between researcher and participant to the social interaction they share' (Sandelowski & Barroso, 2002, p. 216). Banks, et al. (2013) describe reflexivity as a central ethical practice in participatory research where the researcher is 'an embedded participant with situated and partial relationships, responsibilities, values and commitments that frame and constrain ways of seeing, judging and acting in particular situations' (p. 266). Reflexivity is necessary for negotiating the relational and unpredictable power dynamics inherent to participatory research, where community members, researchers and other partners come together to examine and confront issues of disadvantage and marginalisation.

Solidarity as an ethic of action

Feminist participatory researcher, Patricia Maguire (1987), identified solidarity as fundamental to the action-orientation of participatory research, claiming that when the researcher is in solidarity with community members she is not distanced from the struggle for social change; rather she becomes a 'passionate frontline participant in the work to construct a just world' (p. 105). Solidarity is thus highly compatible with the participatory worldview invoking ideas of unity, mutual support, social justice and collective resistance to oppression. Despite these connections, we have found that the term 'solidarity' is seemingly unexamined as a distinct ethical concept in the participatory research field.

In bio-ethics, Prainsack and Buyx (2017), offer a transferable definition of solidarity that we believe could be of use in participatory research. They define solidarity as 'an enacted commitment to carry "costs" (financial, social, emotional or otherwise) to assist others with whom a person or persons recognise similarity in a relevant respect' (p. 52). The phrase 'similarity in a relevant respect' does not necessarily entail shared lived experience; rather, it is a bond that makes it possible to willingly shoulder costs and offer support through action (Prainsack & Buyx, 2017). In other words, solidarity is not built on homogeneity but rather from our relational duties to each other, even across difference, as we share a common purpose and demonstrate commitment through action.

Other authors in philosophy, psychology and theology provide similar definitions of solidarity, noting the importance of understanding context; recognising commonality, interpersonal bonds and interdependence; and demonstrating a readiness to carry costs, sacrifices or burdens for others through action (Sangiovanni, 2015: Laitinen & Pessi, 2014; Brown, 2013). Importantly, according to these authors, solidarity is also linked to collective practices that critique the social order and take action against the harms of injustice. This provokes a fundamental question researchers must ask themselves about their motivation to use a participatory research approach: for what purpose are we seeking to understand the pain of those who suffer the social and health disadvantages of oppression, if not to join in solidarity with them and do something about it?

Examining power through a framework of reflexive-solidarity

Solidarity requires a willingness to carry costs, yet as discussed in our earlier examination of power, the costs for researchers, community members, and other stakeholders will differ greatly in participatory research contexts. A reflexive consideration of solidarity must recognise that people will come to the research with different privileges and opportunities, and bear the costs of their engagement in vastly different ways. This is powerfully illustrated in Case 8.1 where academic researchers in the Netherlands try to stimulate social action among very isolated women and find that efforts to further engage policy-makers results in disappointment.

A failure to be reflexive about power can result in perpetuating unexamined biases and exploitation, thus reinforcing, rather than challenging, systemic oppression (Brown, 2013). Common ethical concepts in participatory research (such as trust, respect, reciprocity and beneficence) are important as a matter of ensuring that community members are not harmed in the process of their engagement; however, solidarity goes further by making explicit that those in relatively powerful positions (such as professional researchers, funders, services providers and policy-makers) have a responsibility to critically examine power relations and share the costs of challenging disadvantage through their own commitments to action. Solidarity does not allow for the onus for action to sit on the shoulders of community members alone; rather, this responsibility must be shared in order to shift from individual/ group level change toward broader sustainable structural and systemic change.

The costs carried by the relatively powerful will vary depending on their role: whether an academic or community based researcher; a community leader with a louder, stronger voice; the decision maker funding a research project; or the institutional power-holders driving the research impact agenda. Across the board, however, these costs will often come down to giving up some level of power and control over the research process and finding ways to take action that are in solidarity with the actions of community members themselves. For researchers, this will include taking up actions that extend beyond traditional research outputs, even when institutions do not value or support community-based work as part of the researchers' role (Stoecker, 1999; Cancian, 1993). While action in solidarity may include academic outputs such as publications, public speaking, and networking, there are certainly other actions that participatory researchers could perform as a matter of sharing the responsibility for progressing social change goals with community partners. For example, this may include: offering support and resources for individual/group-led social action; providing platforms through which community voices can be heard; applying for further funding to help sustain momentum for action and change; and advocating to policy-makers, legislators and other power-holders.

Implementing reflexive-solidarity through dialogue

Most importantly, implementing a reflexive-solidarity framework is not a solitary exercise. It requires continuous and open dialogue amongst researchers, community members, and other allies. Case 8.4, for example, illustrates the importance of reflexive dialogue with community members as part of the change-making process. Dialogue is critical for considering the risks and benefits of action within socio-political contexts; examining the dynamics and impacts of power; and testing ideas about various forms of action and shared social change goals. Reflexive dialogue about solidarity-based action must also ensure that those who hold relative power are taking action in ways that will not risk bringing further adverse impacts on communities.

In the next section, four case studies are presented and analysed to consider how a reflexive-solidarity framework may be applied practically to the action and social change challenges participatory researchers face in various research contexts. These case studies are drawn from the experiences of academic and community-based researchers involved in participatory research projects in the Netherlands, the Philippines, South Africa and Australia. Despite the diversity of these cases and their geographic settings, the authors describe many of the same concerns about responsibilities for action, contributing to broader social change outcomes, and working with complex power dynamics.

PART 2: CASES AND COMMENTARIES

Case 8.1 Striving for social change through participatory research: Challenges in working in a multi-ethnic neighbourhood in the Netherlands

Saskia Duijs and Vivianne Baur

Introduction

This case study is written by a PhD student and a postdoctoral researcher undertaking participatory research in the Netherlands. The political context of the project was characterised by welfare retrenchments due to the financial crisis, enforcement of the Social Support Act (Wet Maatschappelijke Ondersteuning, WMO) and decentralisation of welfare services from the national government to local municipalities. At that time, local government policies aimed to foster citizen participation as an alternative to formal and professional care arrangements.

The case

A participatory research project was established in a relatively poor urban neighbourhood to study and support citizen participation through collective action and reflection. This neighbourhood was considered multi-ethnic by local policy-makers and neighbourhood citizens, as 25 per cent of residents had a non-western background (compared to a city average of 10 per cent), mainly with Moroccan or Turkish roots. This project was funded by a local elderly care organisation and carried out by an all-white Dutch academic research team comprising a doctoral researcher (Duijs), a post-doctoral researcher (Baur) and a professor (also the PhD supervisor). The local elderly care organisation was part of a neighbourhood platform of professional care organisations, established by the local government at the time of our research, to support citizen participation in the neighbourhood. They funded our research to express their support for this platform, but played little role in doing the research. This particular neighbourhood was chosen by the local government because of its high proportion of citizens receiving professional care and low level of citizen participation.

We started our research with a period of ethnographic fieldwork observing community meetings, talking with people on the street and undertaking (informal) interviews with residents. During this period we came into contact with several women who said they wished to get more involved in the neighbourhood. We invited nine women to form an action group to share their experiences, dreams and collaboratively develop ideas and actions for social change, which we facilitated. Our approach was informed by theories of deliberative democracy, enclave deliberation, relational empowerment and collective action. Two women resigned before the project started, but a group of five to seven women regularly met – with eight meetings between March and September 2014. These women came from diverse cultural and religious backgrounds: three were born in Turkey, two fled from Rwanda and Iraq, and two were born and raised within this particular neighbourhood (one Dutch woman who spoke the local dialect and one Indonesian woman). They were aged between 35 and 60. A few had previously been active in their neighbourhood. Yet, most lived very isolated lives, some hardly spoke Dutch and several were struggling to find work. They had few local contacts.

As a research team we aimed to foster social change and citizen participation in this neighbourhood. Yet, during the research process we often struggled with this agenda, as it confronted us with several moral dilemmas. These mainly concerned tensions between striving for social action and social change and acknowledging the vulnerabilities and suffering of the women participating in this participatory research project.

In the early meetings of the action group, the women shared experiences of loneliness, exclusion and discrimination and brought up ideas to promote social contact and informal gatherings with other women in the neighbourhood. The women valued the project for sharing experiences, but although they expressed their wish to promote social contact with other woman locally, they continued sharing their own stories without taking any initiatives to actually organise something. There seemed to be a lack of focus, confidence and shared responsibility to take action. After four or five meetings, we felt we had arrived at a 'dead end'. Together with the supervising professor we decided to adopt an appreciative approach, bearing the words of Mertens (2009) in mind: 'one of the major principles underlying transformative research and evaluation is the belief in the strength that is often overlooked in communities'. We decided to focus on the strengths of these women, hoping this could breathe 'new life' into the action group. Yet, our approach seemed to confront them with the structural exclusion they faced.

During the next meeting one of the women, again, shared her desire for encounters with other women. We asked her: 'What does your dream look like? What is the first step you can take to make this dream possible? What possibilities are already in your reach? Who do you already know and would you like to invite?'

But she bowed her head and remained quiet. Another woman said quietly: 'But we don't know anyone around here.' While another commented about her neighbours: 'No one is ever here, they are always at work or busy doing other things.' We pressed for possibilities: 'Could you approach them in the evening? Or focus on the people who are at home during the day?' Again, the women shared their frustrations and doubts, this time more forcefully: 'Listen, we don't even know their language.' Some expressed shame toward their neighbours and referred to their cultural background and inability to speak the language: 'I cannot imagine myself . . . going up there ringing their doorbell? What will they think of me?' The harder we tried to support these women to take action, through our appreciative approach, the more they expressed frustration and powerlessness. They didn't see any possibilities to connect with other residents and felt ashamed even to consider trying to reach out.

We wondered: what should we do as participatory researchers during this meeting? Should we persist in our appreciative approach to foster collective action, feeling as if we were ignoring the pain and struggles of the women's daily reality? Or should we 'settle' for creating space for sharing stories, with the risk of never doing anything? This question puzzled us long after the project ended. How much space is there for suffering and vulnerability in participatory research aimed at social action and social change? Although giving voice to the perspectives and concerns of these women was at the heart of our approach, we also wanted to foster social action. This moment in our research made us realise that this balance is not easily found.

Looking back, we realise our social change agenda was informed by current policy discourses on 'citizen participation'. Yet, during this project our perspective changed from fostering citizen participation to advocacy on behalf of the women. We felt increasingly compelled to strive for the acknowledgement of the difficulties they faced in organising themselves, due to their own vulnerabilities or mechanisms of structural exclusion. Later in this project we organised a meeting with local policy-makers. Yet, in this meeting the women did not feel heard. Also in other meetings with policy-makers or professionals, the stories of these women did not foster dialogue on the ideal of citizen participation. Local policy seemed to be beyond debate and we felt confronted by our inability as researchers and neighbourhood residents to have a voice in these developments.

So, if there was no room for the women's voices within the given political context, should we keep on motivating them to be part of our project that aimed, against all odds, at social action and social change? To what extent was it our responsibility to protect these women from participating in a project, which appeared to become a disempowering enterprise? For us, this project also raised questions about what is 'social action' and whose agenda is leading when we aim for 'social change'?

Commentary on Case 8.1

Erin Davis and Cathy Vaughan

In this case study, institutional (university, government) bodies implemented a participatory research project aiming to increase citizen participation in a multicultural, economically disadvantaged urban neighbourhood. Outcomes were centred on finding ways for a group of women from diverse cultural backgrounds to undertake actions that would increase their social contact with other women in the neighbourhood. The authors identified the ethical dilemma wherein the capacity of the women to take action was hindered by the very structural barriers that the research engagement was intended to address. Furthermore, this research was situated in a broader context in which 'citizens' were expected to take responsibility to address structural disadvantage brought about by government decentralisation of welfare services.

The women in this project faced isolation and language barriers, as well as fears and vulnerabilities that prevented them from taking on suggested actions such as approaching neighbours or organising a local event. The authors remark that expectations for taking action were placed on the women themselves, and when this did not eventuate, it appeared as though the women were responsible for failing to change the structural barriers shaping their circumstances. Often participatory research projects aim to foster 'citizen action', and yet of all agents involved, disadvantaged citizens may be those with the least resources, capacity and power to take meaningful action. The researchers attempted to address this through advocacy to policy-makers, suggesting a direct dialogue with the women. This too exposed the structural barriers at play as the women were left unheard and disempowered by their meeting with those who had greater capacity to effect change at a broader level. This raises questions about how social change agendas are set and where the responsibility for action lies.

The authors describe a dialogical process when they first met with the women to explore their interests in citizen engagement. Perhaps an overtly reflexive-solidarity approach might assist to also identify the structural barriers and power dynamics impacting on the women's expectations and desires for change. This may present opportunities much earlier in the research project to devise collective responsibilities for action among community members, researchers, funders, and policy-makers.

By reflecting upon these contexts with community members, participatory researchers can identify what supports might be needed for realisation of some 'small wins' (Scheyvens, 1998) and avoid setting expectations that disadvantaged migrant women can transform structural inequality. For example, dialogue in solidarity with community members could produce a plan whereby the researchers 'test the waters' for change by taking their own actions to meet with policy-makers or do some door knocking themselves to explore opportunities for neighbourhood connections. Researchers could then report back on the outcomes and plan new strategies and actions with community members that they might collectively undertake to push for change.

Case 8.2 Shaking things up: participatory research with women with disabilities in the Philippines

Raquel Ignacio

Introduction

This case is written from my perspective as a community organiser and activist with a long history of engagement in the women's movement in the Philippines. It is about a participatory research project on the sexual and reproductive health of women with disabilities, based on collaboration between universities and non-government organisations. The project took place at a time of polarised debate around reproductive health rights in the Philippines.

The case

I worked for a local university in the area of women's rights, and became involved in a participatory research project on the sexual and reproductive health of women with disabilities in the Philippines. The project team was made up of representatives from organisations of people with disabilities, researchers from academic institutions, and advocates from a non-government organisation providing reproductive health services.

Baseline data collection identified various barriers to sexual and reproductive health for women with disabilities, and pilot interventions or 'actions' were developed in response. One of these was the formation and support of peer support groups for women with disabilities, known as PAGs (Participatory Action Groups), which aimed to facilitate access to sexual and reproductive health services for women with disabilities. Five groups were formed (one group of women who are deaf and hard of hearing, one group of women who are blind or have low vision, and three groups of women with mobility impairments). Each team was composed of eight to ten women; however, the group of women who are deaf and hard of hearing had 16 members. The participants were recruited through the assistance of barangay workers (barangays are the smallest unit of government in the Philippines), schools and disability organisations. The majority of the participants were unemployed, still living with and financially dependent upon their parents. The majority of the women had had limited access to education, with only a few having finished (or still in) college. Most of the PAG participants were not involved in any community-based organisations or people with disabilities organisations, and experienced varying degrees of social isolation.

The PAG intervention involved a series of ten peer-facilitated meetings that were held about every fortnight over a 20-week period, with each meeting lasting between a half and a full day. I coordinated the intervention, supporting and mentoring the peer-facilitators, and ensuring that the complex logistical arrangements required to bring women with disabilities together were in place.

The PAG sessions focused on various topics related to sexual and reproductive health and disability, such as the rights of people with disabilities; sexual health and care; pregnancy, family planning and reproductive rights; safety and preventing violence. The women completed a survey before and after the intervention, and participated in interviews upon completion of the ten meetings, to measure changes in their knowledge and practices in relation to sexual and reproductive health. Some women also participated in a follow up interview nine months after the intervention was completed, to assess whether or not changes had been sustained, and to explore other change or opportunities that the participants attributed to the PAGs.

The intervention resulted in a substantial increase in the women's knowledge about sexual and reproductive health, and there were participants who accessed family planning and other sexual and reproductive health services, and violence response services, for the first time. The PAG participants treasured the friendships they had built with their fellow participants and many of them stayed in touch even after the project ended. Many of them reported that gaining self-confidence was a significant result of their participation in the PAG.

I think the PAG sessions presented a lot of possibilities for women with disabilities. The PAG sessions made the women want to continue to be involved in activities where they can mingle with other women with disabilities, learn more about their rights as women and people with disabilities, be exposed to other groups such as local government, disabled people's organisations and civil society organisations. The women want to continue what they have started in PAG.

However, I feel that the project did not sufficiently plan how to sustain the gains of PAGs. The project supported the PAGs to establish links with local disabled people's organisations and local government personnel, anticipating that local organisations would be the right 'home' for the PAGs in future. Though there are five participants who have been able to join in with existing disabled people's organisations, the majority of the women have not and are still waiting for any upcoming PAG activities, even though none are planned. Barriers such as the lack of accessible transport, communication barriers, poverty and gender inequality make it very difficult for women with disabilities to join existing groups. We knew these factors were a barrier to health and other services, and probably should have recognised how difficult it would be for women to participate in the community without extensive supports, even at the local level.

I feel that this means there was a disservice to women with disabilities. It is like we took a bottle of water, shook it up and created bubbles, and now we have just left it alone. But the bubbles do not disappear straight away. The PAG activities made the women think that they can do more – for themselves and for their fellow women with disabilities despite their disabilities. Because there was no programme in place that will continue the initiatives of the research project, the women are left hanging. I wonder about responsibility for sustaining social action that starts during participatory research. Projects shake things up, but projects will always come to an end at some stage – where does responsibility lie for keeping social action moving?

Commentary on Case 8.2

Erin Davis and Cathy Vaughan

This case study shows how the psychosocial benefits of participatory research motivate individual or group led social action, yet these benefits can be undermined by unsustainable resourcing and a lack of clear responsibilities to maintain the momentum of further action toward collective social change goals.

Through their collaborative involvement in knowledge production, participants saw the potential for further improvements in their own lives and the lives of other women with disabilities seeking to access their sexual and reproductive health rights. As in Case 8.1, the women were hindered by the issues of structural inequality that isolated them from each other in the first place and left them bearing the costs of taking further action. The limited resources available for participants to maintain connections and continue social action together made it evident that participatory research projects can both create and then restrict opportunities for change.

The answer to this problem may be partly resolved by the institutional provision of more funding and longer periods of engagement in participatory research projects. Even with the dispensation of greater resources, however, eventually projects do come to an end one way or another. Nevertheless, unlike more conventional research approaches, participatory research fosters opportunities for solidarity building as community members share their experiences, knowledge and desires for social change together. This presents an opportunity for researchers and community members to reflexively dialogue about the scope and limitations of their actions; how to face the realities of funding and time limitations head on; and devise creative and shared strategies for sustainability. Solidarity work may include making agreements about the types of actions necessary to continue striving towards social change goals, but also identifying local resources and champions who can help take the lead on meeting the practical requirements of ongoing action before the research project comes to its inevitable conclusion. Such champions may come from the original research engagement or there may be a need to connect community participants with allies in organisations or activist groups who are already engaged in relevant social change movements.

Case 8.3 Research for social change: Developing understandings of conflicts between conservation and rural livelihoods in Kosi Bay, South Africa

Philile Mbatha

Introduction

This case is written by a South African PhD student, who undertook participatory research in the Kosi Bay area of KwaZulu Natal, an ecologically unique area of interlinked lakes, consisting of five different ecological systems: dune forests, sandy beaches, rich tidal and coral reef zones, as well as grasslands. The local people weave their livelihoods around these resources, and engage in activities such as agriculture, fisheries, forestry and eco-tourism. The communities of Kosi Bay exist in the midst of a myriad of overlapping and conflicting governance arrangements at international and local levels for resource conservation, including the iSimangaliso UNESCO World Heritage Site. This creates confusion on the ground and impacts the conditions for taking action and expectations for social change.

The case

Research for my PhD focused on the tensions between requirements for conservation and the need for local inhabitants to make a living in the impoverished rural area of Kosi Bay. The aim was to understand how indigenous people's livelihood strategies are influenced by the existing governing systems. I adopted an action research approach, as it had always been a passion of mine to conduct research that would bring about policy improvements that could change the lives of people residing in marginalised rural coastal environments in South Africa. It also had a participatory element as I involved some local people as researchers.

Conducting participatory research in Kosi Bay has been fundamentally challenging because coastal conservation is tied to a history of marginalisation, dispossession and exclusion of local people's rights of access to and use of coastal resources. This includes rights of access to fishing, agriculture, harvesting of timber and non-timber forest products, as well as other historical livelihoods that have been undermined by conservation interventions, especially since the advent of the apartheid era in 1948. Most research in Kosi Bay, especially between the 1960s and the 2000, focused on ecological aspects of natural resource systems (particularly fisheries).

On my pilot visit, I obtained permission from both the chief and headman to conduct my research. Community leaders had informed me that obtaining the permission of the chief and headman was adequate for me to proceed with the research. However, upon arriving in one of the villages (Nkovukeni village) for the first time after the research was introduced to the traditional authorities, some community members were outraged when they saw me and my field assistants visiting individual homesteads to pilot the household questionnaire. There appeared to be general consensus among village members that the research could not continue until a village level meeting was called by myself to explain the purpose of the research and gain formal consent from the villagers themselves. When I explained to the people of Nkovukeni that the required permission to conduct the research had been obtained, they insisted that they did not recognise such permission. They felt that the traditional authorities have not prioritised the needs of the people in their village over the years, and they no longer recognised the decisions made by these authorities on behalf of the village. It then became clear to me that although people in different villages of Kosi Bay fall under the same leadership, they are still very divided in some aspects.

I therefore welcomed the request and another meeting was held where I explained the research objectives. At this meeting, people expressed how marginalised they felt in terms of decision-making processes, especially those related to land and distribution of benefits from coastal resources and conservation. They also said they had become skeptical of researchers coming into the area, because researchers never provide feedback about the research that they conduct and usually use their research to inform laws that end up undermining the livelihoods of local people. They even expressed how troubled the word 'research' made them feel, as during colonial and apartheid eras, their land and resources were taken away from them under the guise of research, and ever since they do not trust researchers.

I had to carefully explain the objectives of this research. After discussing the objectives, people said they appreciated this type of research that included them because often researchers have come into the area to research plants, forests and fish, but ignored the people living in the area. Therefore, after a few days, I was informed that people would welcome the research and would appreciate me sharing the findings at the end, and also assisting village members to better understand national and international policies and legislation about conservation that were affecting them.

The research was thus conducted in a participatory manner, ensuring that the communities benefited. Local community assistants were employed to assist with data collection. I also conducted ethnographic research while I resided within the communities for a period of up to five months and was hosted by one of the families in the villages as a way of giving back and also building trust with local people. The findings of this research have been constantly fed back to the communities, as well as other actors involved in the governance, so as to contribute towards improving the livelihoods of people through better decision-making processes.

Through conducting various oral history interviews, focus group meetings, transect walks and ethnographic data collection exercises, I was able to unearth some of the deep grievances of the communities about coastal governance, which they never had the platform to express in this way before. Participating in the research gave the community a voice for the first time. However, this caused me some concerns, as I realised I had unintentionally raised expectations for social change that were beyond the scope of the research. Many community members said the research gave them hope that policy processes that have undermined them for many years would eventually be challenged through the research findings and recommendations. Although I am very passionate about conducting research that would result in social change, I was also aware of the constraints on my capacity as a young researcher to bridge the gap between this marginalised community and policy-makers who sit at the top and are ignorant about realities on the ground.

However, I found that as a researcher one has to be always aware of the role one plays as an academic and at the same time a possible agent of change. Educating the Kosi Bay community about their constitutional rights, as well as using resources available to me to assist community members to participate in policy decision platforms that they are not usually invited to, has empowered the community to use the research to challenge policy-makers on their own. What was also pivotal in this process was the fact that many of the policies affecting this community's rights are not written in their indigenous language (i.e. isiZulu). It was therefore difficult for local people to understand these pieces of legislation. Through the research, the community became empowered as they began to understand different laws and policies that affect them, so that they can effectively participate in decision-making platforms when the opportunity arises.

Commentary on Case 8.3

Erin Davis and Cathy Vaughan

In this case, community members themselves highlighted the importance of a soli-darity ethic when they questioned the validity of the chief and headman's authori-sation of the research and expressed concerns about previous research projects that undermined their rights and agency. In doing so, they demonstrated how they were already engaging in their own critically conscious actions to resist power-over dynamics and improve their social and political conditions.

Reflexivity is necessary to identify top-down approaches that rely too heavily on authorisation by outsiders or those who hold gatekeeping status over a com-munity. This can negatively impact action and social change arising from partici-patory research, as community members are unable to take control of the means of producing, distributing and acting on knowledge about themselves and the issues that affect them. A reflexive-solidarity framework considers complex institutional and community-based power dynamics in order to more effectively progress participation and action towards social change goals derived from the interests of community members themselves. This is seen when the author describes how she overcame the initial hurdles with engagement and came to act through a solidarity ethic by placing community members into positions of research ownership that would serve their grassroots activism.

Interestingly, as action outcomes began to take shape, the author became con-cerned about whether the project would meet community members' expectations for social change. This is also expressed in Case 8.2, where unsustained resources hindered momentum towards change leaving community members disappointed that they may not be able to continue with their social action efforts.

It seems that when participatory research projects are successfully participatory and action-oriented, the concern about whether or not actions are adequate and whether social change is actually possible begins to plague those involved. We think it is important to recognise that this is not a concern unique to participatory researchers. As discussed in Part 1, social change is a long and convoluted process fed by numerous actions and movements, of which participatory research is just one of many contributors. A reflexive-solidarity framework can be enacted to transparently engage community members about the realistic outcomes they would expect from a participatory research project and link the contributory actions of participatory research to broader social change movements. This case study gives some insights into this process as the activist foundations laid by the community members themselves, and supported through the solidarity-based actions of the researcher, created opportunities for the research project to have a positive impact on the wider community.

Case 8.4 Researching community-led responses to family violence in Australia: Whose vision of socially just change?

Jasmin Chen

Introduction

This case is written by a research assistant from a feminist multicultural women's health organisation in Melbourne, Australia. The case describes a participatory research project that investigated immigrant and refugee women's experiences of domestic violence as well as community-led and systemic responses to the issue. The author describes an ethical dilemma when discovering that a community member involved with the project did not seem to share her organisation's feminist values, thus challenging assumptions about a shared basis for social change.

The case

I am a research assistant at the Multicultural Centre for Women's Health (MCWH). To work at MCWH is to share in and build on a proud immigrant feminist legacy. For over 40 years, our organisation has been run by and for immigrant and refugee women to improve women's health through education and leadership. Our approach is founded on respecting and strengthening immigrant and refugee women's voices, choices and expertise.

While the core of our work involves offering women bilingual peer education and information about their health and rights, we also advocate for change. We call for governments to address structural and systemic issues that undermine immigrant women's health. We highlight ways immigrant women are one-dimensionally represented and treated in mainstream contexts. Most importantly, we argue that immigrant and refugee communities in general, and women in particular, should be equal partners and leaders in decision making about their own health and well-being.

In our advocacy, we have often found our greatest challenge to be the absence of a reliable evidence-base to support our positions and programmes. For the last five years we have been actively seeking researchers who are interested in undertaking research to substantiate our position and share our vision and values. When we encountered participatory research, with its explicit objective of social change, we felt that it was a perfect fit. It is an approach that endorses our belief that social change must be driven and led by those directly affected.

We were funded to conduct a participatory research project on 'community-led responses to family violence' in partnership with a group of academic researchers with whom we had established a previous relationship. Our partnership was not just collaboration between a community organisation and university academics, where our roles remained quite separate. Rather, three employees of our organisation were integral co-investigators, and contributed to all aspects of the research, from beginning to end. The research funding was split between our organisation and the university.

Although the project was ambitious in scope, our organisation drew confidence from the knowledge that, whatever our findings, they would be framed by our research team's shared aims for social justice. We knew from the outset that the research design would align with our ethics; that the research process would not exploit, undermine or distort immigrant and refugee women's experiences or views. We knew, and still know, that the research team shared our commitment to improving the health and well-being of women. Although at the time I took it for granted, our trust that the research team shared our vision for social change was integral to our confidence in the research process.

We felt a strong responsibility to represent in our findings the diverse views and experiences of a broad range of women and groups, from a wide range of communities and regions. Our approach was intersectional and feminist, and throughout the project we went to every effort to engage groups of different ages, stages of migration and life, religious identities, visa types and countries of birth. The research team often reaffirmed our commitment to women's voices, community leadership and community-led expertise. Parts of the research that I was closely involved in allowed me to build relationships with women who had experienced violence and had ideas for change. I supported a group of women using visual methods to communicate their perspectives in more than words. The process of working with this group, in particular, seemed to exemplify participatory research and what it represents methodologically (at least as I understand it). With these women we were jointly producing new understandings about responding to and preventing family violence in immigrant and refugee communities. The group spoke at length about the gaps in current family violence support for women, about their vision for better responses and their hopes for women in the future. Yet, not all of these women's ideas aligned with our vision for social change as an organisation. Several ideas stood in opposition to our 'feminist' principles, and one woman's suggestions indicated a classist attitude to members of the same ethno-specific community.

One evening, I was driving home with one of the group members, a woman leading responses to violence in her community and who played a leadership role within the visual methods group. During our conversation, I felt challenged by her remark that a woman should have the 'common sense' to know that when her husband comes home drunk, it's not a good time to start an argument. I felt confused about how to respond. As a researcher I felt I should regard her view as relevant data. As an advocate, I felt I should question her position, maybe even dispute it. But at that moment, I questioned whether participatory research really allowed me to be both. I chose to gently question her view, not as a researcher but as an advocate, or maybe not even as that: perhaps as a woman who had finished for the day and was driving a friend home. I wondered though, after the car ride was over, what it would mean if the 'community-led responses' that the women we were working with came up with did not fit with our ideas about appropriate social action, our approach or our values.

Here is the problem then. Is it our right as researchers to set the terms of social action? What happens when what the community has to say does not align with your vision of social change? How do we, as researchers, balance our fidelity to what community members say with our own ethics, when what is at stake is the shape and character of the social action to be undertaken? How do we do this as participatory researchers, who claim to value the expertise, knowledge and authority of communities as much as that of formally trained researchers? What does it mean to enter into research with an explicit motivation for a specific type of social change? Does participatory research assume that social change will always be in the interests of the community, regardless of what the community says? Social change is not benign, but highly active. It is not politically neutral. Does the assumption underlying most participatory research definitions of social change link it to social justice and 'left' politics? What happens when someone's ideas about social change look 'right' instead?

The number of women we spoke to who shared our vision far outweighed those few voices that challenged our view. However, to be representative of the qualitative outcomes from our research, our research team described nuances in community views and were faithful to immigrant and refugee women's words and intentions. Our research did not waver from that ethical responsibility and I am proud to have been part of it. But what happens to participatory action when views about social change are at odds? What is our obligation as community-based or academic researchers to honour these views?

Commentary on Case 8.4

Erin Davis and Cathy Vaughan

Here we have a case study that challenges assumptions about solidarity. Reflexivity is important here, in particular the kind of dialogical reflexivity that takes a critical approach and faces up to conflict in the research context. Indeed, conflict cannot be avoided in the inherently relational and power-laden dynamics of participatory research. This is evident as this case highlights the interplay of power, gender, culture and class. Such complexities will inevitably result in conflicting ideas about the issues at stake and how to handle them.

The author discusses the difficulties in finding that a community leader expressed a view that was in conflict with the intersectional feminist approach that underpinned the research project they were engaged in together. To avoid what was likely a difficult conversation, the author could have chosen to not say anything at all in response to the community member's remarks. Yet, she chose to engage in a critically reflexive dialogue in that moment. Knowledge was co-constructed in this conversation, even if it presented challenges and did not lead to any particular resolution at that time.

These difficult conversations are part of engaging in a reflexive-solidarity framework and testing assumptions about our shared purpose for action and social change. Perhaps a reflexive dialogue with community members as a group from the start of the project would help in this regard, at least to identify these issues early and navigate through them along the way. This may also require that these early conversations involve discussions about the foundational values that underpin collective understanding of the issues being researched and how this might influence participants' visions of action and social change. In this case, the author described the importance of an intersectional feminist lens to the research project and engaged with this lens in her discussion with the community member.

As in Case 8.3, this situation exemplifies the kind of power relations within communities that can inhibit social change, where those who are in relatively more powerful positions hold views that could potentially be damaging to those in the community who are more affected by the issues being researched. The author is aware of the community member's powerful position in this regard, but also considers her own role as a researcher to honour community-led views. This in itself demonstrates a reflexive-solidarity approach as the researcher examines the complexities of power impacting on the research project.

We suggest that the author's concern about imposing her knowledge during the difficult conversation might be assuaged by considering how she acted in solidarity through honouring the experiences of the many other women she encountered in the project and also in her everyday work within a community organisation that advocates for immigrant and refugee women's rights. This is not a matter of disregarding the individual community member's point of view, but rather to engage with her in dialogue about those views while considering how they might affect bigger social change efforts in relation to violence against women. Solidarity work is not easy, but social change necessitates that we work through these challenges to move forward and reach new possibilities.

PART 3: CONCLUDING COMMENTS

Erin Davis and Cathy Vaughan

In this chapter we put forth the argument that the theoretical origins, praxis and transformative potential of participatory research necessitates a guiding ethical framework that supports its action-oriented approach and links research contributions to broader social change goals.

We examined how the theoretical underpinnings of a participatory worldview establish action and social change as critical components of participatory research.

Three interrelated concepts of action and social change were explored: 1) individual/group level change (typically affecting those directly involved in research projects); 2) social action arising from the critical consciousness brought about by individual/group level change; and 3) broader social change at systemic and structural levels, whereby participatory research is considered a contributor alongside activist campaigning, advocacy work, and other political and legislative reforms. We considered how action is inhibited by manifestations of institutional and community power dynamics creating ethical dilemmas and tensions for participatory researchers and community members. As such, the action-orientation of participatory research requires a guiding ethical approach, which we describe through a framework drawing on the ethics of reflexivity and solidarity.

A reflexive-solidarity ethical framework involves introspection, open dialogue, and a willingness to take collective responsibility for action. In solidarity, the costs of action should not be carried solely by community members, but also by researchers, community advocates, policy-makers, institutional power holders and others involved in participatory research endeavours. Dialogical reflexivity is necessary to strategise action while examining assumptions about the values and perspectives that inform beliefs about action and social change, and critiquing the institutional and community power dynamics that shape the outcomes of research projects.

The four case studies from the Netherlands, the Philippines, South Africa and Australia, illustrate ethical challenges arising from the action-orientation of participatory research. Applying the reflexive-solidarity framework to these case studies provides an opportunity to examine how researchers can respond to these challenges and engage dialogical reflexivity with community members to: find opportunities to progress and sustain action outcomes; challenge structural and systemic barriers; and join up with relevant social change efforts. These cases also point to similarities in the experiences of participatory researchers, despite their diverse settings. Reducing isolation and identifying commonalities is critical, not only for community members who challenge the effects of oppression through their involvement in research, but also for researchers themselves.

We recognise that the ethical dilemmas arising from the 'action' element of participatory research are challenging and can be difficult to communicate and tangibly address in our work, particularly when compared to more traditional research approaches. This chapter was conceived in a spirit of solidarity with those that seek to utilise research as a contribution to social change and we hope that articulating an ethical framework of reflexivity and solidarity is useful in progressing action from participatory research praxis.

References

Banks, S., Armstrong, A., Carter, K., Graham, H., Hayward, P., Henry, A., . . . Strachan, A. (2013). Everyday ethics in community-based participatory research. *Contemporary Social Science, 8*(3), 263–277.

Banks, S., Herrington, T., & Carter, K. (2017). Pathways to co-impact: action research and community organising. *Educational Action Research, 25*(4), 541–559.

Brown, T. (2013). Realizing a research ethic of solidarity: The role of the unconscious and an ontology drawn from Zen Buddhist teachings on nonduality. *International Journal of Multiple Research Approaches, 7*(3), 374–383.

Cancian, F. (1993). Conflicts between Activist Research and Academic Success: Participatory Research and Alternative Strategies. *The American Sociologist, 24*(1), 92–106.

Caldwell, W.B., Reyes, A.G., Rowe, Z., Weinert, J., & Israel, B.A. (2015). Community Partner Perspectives on Benefits, Challenges, Facilitating Factors, and Lessons Learned from Community-Based Participatory Research Partnerships in Detroit. *Progress in Community Health Partnerships: Research, Education, and Action, 9*(2), 299–311.

Campbell, C., Cornish, F., Gibbs, A., Scott, K. (2010). Heeding the Push from Below: How do social movements persuade the rich to listen to the poor? *Journal of Health Psychology, 15*(7), 962–971.

Castleden, H., Morgan, V.S., & Lamb, C. (2012). "I spent the first year drinking tea": Exploring Canadian university researchers' perspectives on community-based participatory research involving Indigenous peoples. *Canadian Geographer, 56*(2), 160–179.

Chatterton, P., Fuller, D. & Routledge, P. (2007). Relating action to activism: Theoretical and methodological reflections. In S.L. Kindon, R. Pain, & M. Kesby (Eds.), *Participatory action research approaches and methods: Connecting people, participation and place* (pp. 216–222). London: Routledge.

Cornish F. (2006). Empowerment to participate: a case study of participation by Indian sex workers in HIV prevention. *Journal of Community & Applied Social Psychology, 16*, 301–315.

Darby, S. (2017). Making space for co-produced research 'impact': Learning from a participatory action research case study. *Area, 49*(2), 230–237.

Evans, R. (2016). Achieving and evidencing research 'impact'? Tensions and dilemmas from an ethic of care perspective. *Area, 48*(2), 213–221.

Fine, M. (2012). Troubling calls for evidence: A critical race, class and gender analysis of whose evidence counts. *Feminism & Psychology, 22*(1), 3–19.

Foster-Fishman, P., Nowell, B., Deacon Z., Nievar M.A., & McCann P. (2005). Using methods that matter: the impact of reflection, dialogue, and voice. *American Journal of Community Psychology, 36*(3/4), 275–291.

Freire, P. (1970). *Pedagogy of the oppressed*. New York: Bloomsbury.

George, M.A., Daniel, M. & Green, L.W. (2007). Appraising and Funding Participatory Research in Health Promotion. *International Quarterly of Community Health Education, 26*(2), 171–187.

Golob, M.I., & Giles, A.R. (2013). Challenging and transforming power relations within community-based participatory research: the promise of a Foucauldian analysis. *Qualitative Research in Sport, Exercise and Health, 5*(3), 356–372.

Jordan, S. & Kapoor, D. (2016). Re-politicizing participatory action research: unmasking neoliberalism and the illusions of participation. *Educational Action Research, 24*(1), 134–149.

Laitinen, A., & Pessi, A.B. (2014). Solidarity: Theory and Practice. An Introduction. In A. Laitinen & A.B. Pessi (Eds.), *Solidarity: theory and practice* (pp. 1–29). Lanham, MD: Lexington Books.

Ledwith, M., (2007). On being critical: uniting theory and practice through emancipatory action research. *Educational Action Research, 15*(4), 597–611.

Maguire, P. (1987). *Doing participatory research: A feminist approach*. Amherst: Center for International Education, School of Education, University of Massachusetts.

Mertens, D. (2009). *Transformative Research and Evaluation*. New York: The Guildford Press

Minkler, M. (2004). Ethical challenges for the "outside" researcher in CBPR. *Health Education & Behavior: The Official Publication of the Society for Public Health Education, 31*(6), 684–97.

Nygreen, K. (2009). Critical Dilemmas in PAR: Toward a New Theory of Engaged Research for Social Change. *Social Justice, 36*(4), 14–35.

Prainsack, B., & Buyx, A. (2017). What is Solidarity? In B. Prainsack & A. Buyx (Eds.), *Solidarity in Biomedicine and Beyond* (pp. 43–72). Cambridge: Cambridge University Press.

Reason, P., & Bradbury, H. (2006). Introduction: Inquiry and Participation in Search of a World Worthy of Human Aspiration. In P. Reason & H. Bradbury (Eds.), *Handbook of Action Research* (pp. 1–14). London: SAGE Publications.

Reid, C., Tom, A., & Frisby, W. (2006). Finding the "action" in feminist participatory action research. *Action Research, 4*(3), 315–332.

Sandelowski, M. & Barroso, J. (2002). Finding the Findings in Qualitative Studies. *Journal of Nursing Scholarship, 34*(3), 213–219.

Sangiovanni, A. (2015). Solidarity as Joint Action. *Journal Of Applied Philosophy, 32*(4), 340–359.

Scheyvens, R. (1998). Subtle strategies for women's empowerment: Planning for effective development. *Third World Planning Review, 2*(3), 235–253.

Stoecker, R. (1999). Are Academics Irrelevant?: Roles for Scholars in Participatory Research. *The American Behavioral Scientist, 42*(5), 840–854.

Van der Eb, C.W., Peddle, N., Buntin, M., Isenberg, D.H., Duncan, L., Everett, S., . . . Molloy, P. (2004). Community Concerns About Participatory Research. In L. Jason (Ed.), *Participatory community research: theories and methods in action* (pp. 221–226). Washington, DC: American Psychological Association.

Vaughan, C. (2014). Participatory research with youth: Idealising safe social spaces or building transformative links in difficult environments? *Journal of Health Psychology, 19*(1), 184–192.

Vaughan, C., Zayas, J., Marella, M., Edmonds, T., Garcia, J., Bisda, K.,. . .Marco, M.J. (2014). 'Doing' Action Research: perspectives on rationale, rhetoric, reality and results. *Development Bulletin, 76*, 22–26.

Wallerstein, N. & Duran, B. (2008). The Theoretical, Historical, and Practice Roots of CBPR. In M. Minkler & N. Wallerstein (Eds.), *Community-based participatory research for health: from process to outcomes* (pp. 25–46). San Francisco: Jossey-Bass.

Yoshihama, M., & Carr, E. S. (2002). Community participation reconsidered: Feminist participatory action research with Hmong women. *Journal of Community Practice, 10*(4), 85–104.

INDEX

Aamjiwnaang First Nation Health and Environment Community 4, 116–17
Abma, T. 22, 24–5, 31–55, 103–30
Aboriginal communities 116–19; guidelines for research with 60; *see also* indigenous communities; native people
abuse 62, 136
academic researchers 15, 17, 19, 25, 31–6; and blurred boundaries 57–61, 63, 76; and co-ownership 104–7, 116, 125; and confidentiality 137, 143, 145, 149; and democratic representation 96, 98–9; and non-academic researchers 109; and power 39–43, 49, 51–2; and social change 189–90, 201–2
Academy of Finland 119
accountability 117, 157
action research (AR) 2–3, 11, 25, 40–2, 60; and co-ownership 119; and confidentiality 138, 152; and democratic representation 83, 86, 89, 98; and points of action 57, 63; and review processes 155, 165, 168, 170–6; and social change 197, 204
active learning 21, 87
activism 3–4, 9, 56–79, 87, 104; and co-ownership 116–17; and confidentiality 134, 138; and social change 184–5, 191, 194, 196, 199–200, 204
Adams, V. 40
advisory groups 6, 139, 143–4, 161
advocacy 70, 77, 104–5, 108, 151–2, 181, 184–5, 189, 192–4, 200–2, 204

Africa 15–16, 32, 58, 104, 113,133, 137
African Programme for Onchocerciasis Control 113
age 5, 21, 67–8, 81, 95–6, 105, 160, 201
agency 86, 104, 109, 135, 152, 170, 199
aggregated data 112, 132, 144–5, 159
aid agencies 82
alienation 35, 108, 169–70
animators 83, 86, 88
anonymity 9–10, 16, 23, 25, 131–54, 159, 175
anthropology 57, 83
apartheid 197–8
applications 8, 37, 148, 165, 167, 171–2
appropriation 103
Arctic 24, 81, 95–7
Aristotle 11, 13
Arnstein, S.R. 104
Asia 181
Asperger's syndrome 24, 32, 38, 43–6
assertive outreach (AO) 173–5
assets 81–2
asylum seekers 62
atma-shakti 87
audiences 21, 23, 86, 104, 108–9, 118, 126, 167
Aumann, K. 60
Australia 4, 16, 25, 32, 146–7, 150, 181–2, 190, 200–4
authenticity 37, 56, 89, 111, 120, 123, 175

authors/authorship 1, 9, 14–18, 20, 25; and blurred boundaries 70, 73, 75; and co-ownership 106, 111, 125; and confidentiality 148–9, 152; and democratic representation 80; and power 38, 48; and social change 193, 199, 202–3
Autism Spectrum Disorder (ASD) 43, 132, 138, 150–2
autonomy 41–3, 87, 148, 157

Bangladesh 24, 80, 86, 88
Banks, S. xxiii, 1–30, 149, 187
Barazangi, N.H. 87, 89
Barnardo's 49–50
Baur, V. 18, 181, 190–3
behavioural sciences 8
Belmont Report 7, 156
Beresford, P. 106–7
best practice 17, 76, 134, 153, 161
Bilfeldt, A. 31, 40–2, 43
Bjeloncikova, M. 80, 97–100
blurred boundaries 6, 9–10, 24, 56–79, 109, 134, 146, 159
Boal's Theatre of the Oppressed 24
Bogotá University 3
Bos, G. 24–5, 103–30
Boucher, L. 130
boundary-spanners/crossers 60
Bradley, C. 155, 165–7
Brear, M. 16, 130, 146–8
Brydon-Miller, M. xxiv, 1–30, 135, 152
budgets 36–7, 43, 49–50, 94–5
bureaucracy 34, 157
Buyx, A. 188

Canada 4, 6, 18, 24–5, 80–1; and co-ownership 104, 116–19, 130; and confidentiality 139, 143–5; and democratic representation 89–92, 95–7; and review processes 156, 164, 170, 181; and social change 181
capacity-building 46–9
Cardol, M. 56
care ethics see ethics of care
care workers 40–3, 52
Carr, E.S. 186
caste 85, 88
casuistry 11–13
Central America 90
Centre for Action Research in Professional Practice (CAARP) 175
Centre for Children and Young People's Participation 49

Centre of Client Experience 32
Centre for Social Justice and Community Action (CSJCA) 4, 8
challenges 22, 34–40, 45, 51, 57; and blurred boundaries 59–63, 74–5, 77; and co-ownership 104, 109, 114, 117–18, 120, 122, 125; and confidentiality 131–2, 134–5, 139, 143–7; and democratic representation 81, 87, 93–4, 97, 100; and review processes 155, 157, 163–4, 173, 176; and social change 183, 185–7, 190, 198–202
Chambers, R. 4
Chatterton, P. 184
Chen, J. 181, 200–3
children see young people
Christianity 13
churches 80, 82, 88–92
citizenship 84–5, 119
civil society 2, 195
class 5, 21, 34, 83–5, 181, 201–2
Cleaver, S. 80, 92–4
clinical trials 105, 166–7
clinicians 144–5
co-inquiry groups 72–3
co-option 5, 103, 106–7, 185
co-ownership 1, 24, 103–30, 157
co-production 6, 56–61, 65, 67, 71–2, 166
co-researchers 4, 9, 18–19, 24–5, 33; and blurred boundaries 58, 67, 69, 71–2; and co-ownership 105, 122–5, 130; and confidentiality 134–5, 137, 146–9, 153; and power 38, 41, 43–6, 52; and review processes 167
co-writing 25, 45, 122–5, 148
codes of ethics 20, 156
coercion 25, 159
collaboration 1, 3–4, 6, 8, 13; and blurred boundaries 58, 61, 67; and co-ownership 105–6, 108, 113–18; and confidentiality 143; and democratic representation 89, 91–2, 94–7; and ethics 18, 20–2; and power 31–55; and review processes 157, 169; and social change 183, 191, 194, 196, 201
collective action 20, 22, 190–2
Colombia 3
colonialism 3, 95, 116, 118, 182, 198
colonisation 103, 106, 116–19, 157, 162
communitarianism 1, 11–13, 87
community 5–7, 9, 186–7, 196–200, 202–4; communities of practice 32, 43, 60; community rights 24, 80–102; community-based health research

112–15; community-university research partnerships 5

Community Advisory Committee 139

community researchers 6, 8–9, 15–17, 19, 24–5; and blurred boundaries 57–64, 66, 69–72, 75; and co-ownership 106, 111; and confidentiality 146–9; and power 33, 38

community-based organisations (CBOs) 82

community-based participatory research (CBPR) 4, 6, 14, 20, 25; and confidentiality 132, 141; and democratic representation 87, 97–8; and power 31, 47; and review processes 155; and social change 181

community-based research (CBR) 4, 9, 17, 24–5, 100, 113, 130, 139, 143–6, 181, 190

compensation 33, 36, 48, 121

confidentiality 9–10, 25, 59, 61, 69, 111, 131–54, 163–4, 175

conflict 6, 9, 24, 34–7, 80–102; and confidentiality 141; conflict management 83; conflict resolution 83; conflict transformation 83, 86, 101; conflicts of interest 25, 158–9; and review processes 175; and social change 186, 196–200, 202

consent 2, 7–9, 25, 67, 89; and co-ownership 130; and confidentiality 132–3, 135–6, 142, 144–5, 148–50, 152–3; and review processes 156, 158, 160, 162–6, 168–70, 174–6; and social change 197

conservation 196–200

constructivism 182

contracts 32, 162

Contreras, A. 80, 89–91

control 105–6, 115, 119, 122, 124, 126, 152, 164, 184–6, 189

Cornish, F. 184

Cottrell, B. 157

counselling 169–70

credit 9, 25, 71, 125, 134, 137, 148, 152

criminalisation 139–41, 162

critical consciousness 182–3, 199, 204

critical theory 95, 182

cultural relativism 82

curriculum issues 101, 123

Czech Republic 6, 24, 81, 97–100

Dalla Lana School of Public Health 143

Dar es Salaam University 3

data collection 14–15, 24, 47, 59, 61–2; and blurred boundaries 64–9, 72, 75; and co-ownership 112–15; and confidentiality

133–7, 139, 141, 143, 147; and data management 163–4; and democratic representation 93; and review processes 158–61, 174–5; and social change 183, 194, 198; and stolen data 130, 141–2

Davis, A. 25, 133, 193

Davis, E. 25, 181–203

De Prinse, K. 130, 143

deficit models 44

deliberation, enclave deliberation 191

democracy 3, 33, 40–2, 59, 91; bourgeois democracy 84; civic democracy 84; and co-ownership 109; deep democracy 85; deliberative democracy 191; democratic representation 5, 9, 20–1, 24, 80–102; knowledge democracy 5; liberal democracy 84; and review processes 174; and social change 185

Denmark 24, 32

deontology 10, 175

Developmental Action Logics 35

dialogue 2, 8, 16, 73, 85; and co-ownership 105, 107, 109, 112; and confidentiality 137; and review processes 175; and social change 189–90, 192–3, 196, 202–4

dilemmas 2, 8, 14–16, 20, 25; and blurred boundaries 57–8, 60–1, 66, 69–71, 75–6; and co-ownership 115–17, 122, 125; and confidentiality 132, 136, 138, 148; and democratic representation 85–6; dilemmas cafés 24; and power 35, 37, 45, 51; and review processes 169, 173–4; and social change 191, 193, 200, 204

diplomacy 35

Disability Studies 70, 107

disabilities, people with 9, 24–5, 32, 44, 46; and blurred boundaries 58, 69–74; and co-ownership 104–6, 122–6; and democratic representation 92, 94; and intellectual disabilities 24–5, 58, 69–73, 104–6, 122–6, 169; and learning disabilities 43; and power 50; and review processes 169; and social change 181–2, 186, 194–6

disclaimers 161, 163

disclosure 38, 109, 111, 132–3, 137–8, 141–2, 144–5, 149, 151–2, 174

discrimination 21, 84–5, 88, 98, 108, 139, 191

dissemination 1, 3, 6, 9, 18; and and power 44; and co-ownership 103–30; and confidentiality 134, 147; and ethics 24; and review processes 164, 175; and social change 183

doctoral students 18–19
documentary films 116–19
Dodson, L. 38
domination models 33
Downie, J. 157
Drug use 68, 96, 139–42, 144–6, 161, 164, 173–6
Duchenne parent project 105
Duijs, S. 18, 181, 190–3
Durham Community Research Team 6
Durham University 4, 8, 14
Dutch language 123–5, 191–2

Easter, M. 133
ecology 16, 95, 196–7
ecosystems 10
egalitarian models 33, 51–2, 185
elders 24, 32, 92–3, 117, 190
elites 82, 84
emic knowledge 56
empowerment 3, 39, 70, 81–2, 95; and co-ownership 111; and confidentiality 135, 137–8, 147, 149; and democratic representation 100; and social change 184, 191–2, 198–9
England 43, 49, 58, 174
English language 15–16, 64–5, 124–5
entrepreneurs 105
environment 116–19
epistemology 17, 48, 106, 174
Ethical Review Panels (ERP) 168–70, 173–4, 176; *see also* Institutional Review Boards; Research Ethics Committees/ Boards
ethics 1, 4, 7–13, 57–8, 60; and anonymity 131–54; care ethics 11–13, case-based ethics 11–13; and challenges 60–3; and co-ownership 103–30; and community research 59–60; and community rights 80–102; and confidentiality 131–54; and conflict 80–102; contractual ethics 59–60; covenantal ethics 1, 11, 60, 77; and democratic representation 80–102; and dissemination 103–30; ethical framework 187–90; ethical stance 35, 60; ethics creep 157; ethics work 20; everyday ethics 1, 11, 13, 20, 60, 126, 149; and impact 103–30; and insensitivity to feelings 66; and nature of cases 14–19; narrative ethics 12; in participatory research 1–30; and practice framework 20–2; principle-based ethics 11–13; and privacy 131–54; and research ethics industry 156; and review processes 1, 8–9, 19, 22, 25, 35,

75–7, 113–15, 135, 137–8, 149, 153, 155–80; and sensitivity to feelings 64–6; and social change 181–203; theoretical approaches to 10–14; virtue ethics 1, 11–13; utilitarian ethics, 11-13
ethnicity 5–6, 21, 25, 81, 83, 95, 97–100, 190–3, 201
ethnography 18, 58, 69, 104, 135, 147–8, 191, 198
eugenics 156
Europe 104, 165
European Court of Human Rights 98
evaluation 2, 5, 13–16, 62, 71, 74, 86, 89, 104, 122, 143, 191
exclusion 9, 24, 81, 84–5, 93; and co-ownership 118, 122, 125; and confidentiality 144; and democratic representation 97–100; and review processes 160–1, 174–5; and social change 186, 191–2, 197; *see also* social exclusion
experts/expertise 8, 21, 31–2, 38, 40–2; and blurred boundaries 67, 72; and co-ownership 106, 117, 120, 123; and confidentiality 137, 146; and democratic representation 81–2, 99; and power 48; and review processes 157, 166–7, 170, 176; and social change 182, 200–2
exploitation 8, 90, 201

Facebook 67
facilitators/facilitation 24, 33–7, 48–9, 67, 83, 91, 113–14, 144, 146, 174, 194
Fals Borda, O. 3
fascism 83
feedback 50, 115, 144, 147, 151, 168, 173, 198
feminism 4, 11, 19, 35, 60, 80, 86–7, 92, 95, 182, 188, 200–3
feudalism 84
Fieldhouse, J. 155, 173–6
financial crisis 190
findings 1, 9, 18, 25, 63; and blurred boundaries 67; and co-ownership 110, 112–15, 117; and confidentiality 134–5, 138, 144; and review processes 174; and social change 185, 198, 201
Finland 25, 104, 119–22
First Nations 4, 104, 116–19
Flicker, S. 62
focus groups 44, 47, 67, 69, 71–2, 92, 113–15, 119–20, 160, 168–70, 198
follow-up 67, 91, 121, 140, 172, 174
foreign workers, Temporary Foreign Workers (TFWs) 80, 88–92

Foster-Fishman, P. 184
Freire, P. 3, 182
friendship 9, 17–19, 24, 43, 58; and blurred boundaries 61, 66–72; and co-ownership 120, 126; and confidentiality 133; and democratic representation 96; and social change 195, 202
Fuller, D. 184
funding 35–7, 39, 46–9, 70, 73; and co-ownership 110, 112, 114, 117, 119, 123; and confidentiality 137, 140, 147–9; and review processes 161–2, 174; and social change 186, 189, 191, 193, 196, 201
future research 88, 94, 100, 115, 118; and co-ownership 121, 124–6; and confidentiality 140–2, 144, 148–9; and review processes 160, 166, 173, 176; and social change 183

gatekeepers 186, 199
gender 5, 21, 24, 34, 46–9, 81–2, 85, 95–6, 195, 202
gender-based violence (GBV) 46–9
general practitioners (GPs) 62, 165
George, M.A. 183
Germany 7, 82
Gillard, S. 107
Gilligan, C. 115
Gojova, V. 80, 97–100
good practice 20, 72
governance 8, 60, 174, 197–8
grammar 109, 123–4
grassroots action 82, 117, 147, 182, 199
Greene, S. 61
Greenwood, D. 135, 152
Groot, B. 22, 24, 31–55
Guhathakurta, M. 24, 80–102
guidelines 72, 108, 155–6, 161, 183
Gumplowicz, L. 83
Guta, A. 25, 130, 143, 155–80

Habermas, J. 34
Haggerty, K.D. 157
Hall, B. 3
Hanoi Club 151
haram 88
Hart, A. 60
Health Canada 95
Health, Department of, 174
health care 25, 42–3, 58, 63, 73, 103, 108, 165, 169, 173
health, public 143
health research 1, 4, 7–8, 14, 35; and blurred boundaries 58–60, 64–6, 70;

and co-ownership 104, 111–15; and confidentiality 146–9; and review processes 165, 170–4
Health Research Authority (HRA) 174
hegemony 84
Helsinki Declaration 7, 156
Henderson, G. 133
hepatitis C 139–41
hermeneutics 39, 106; Creative Critical Hermeneutic Analysis 39
Highlander Research and Education Center 4
Hilsen, A.I. 11
Hinduism 88
HIV 64, 133, 139, 143–5, 156
homework 74
hospitals 24, 73–6, 130, 143–5, 156, 168–71, 173–4
housing 82, 98–9, 139
human rights 82, 89–92, 156
Hynes, G. 19, 56, 73–5, 155

identities 4–5, 9, 12, 21, 23; and blurred boundaries 56–60, 63, 66, 72, 75–6; and confidentiality 132, 135–6, 141, 148, 151; and democratic representation 85, 87; and review processes 159; and social change 201
ideology 84, 130, 133, 137
Ignacio, R. 181, 194–6
impact 1–2, 9–10, 24–5, 34, 36; and blurred boundaries 57–8, 63, 74, 76; and co-ownership 103–30; and confidentiality 134, 138, 140–2, 145; and democratic representation 85–7, 91, 93–4; and power 38–9, 48, 52; and review processes 175; and social change 182, 184–7, 189–90, 193, 197, 199–200, 203; understanding change 110
implementation 39–40, 59, 62, 69, 98; and co-ownership 104, 119; and confidentiality 134, 138, 147, 149; and review processes 165, 171, 174; and social change 183, 189–90, 193
India 3
Indigenous communities 4, 11, 16, 18, 60, 95–7, 104, 108, 116–19, 162–4, 197, 199; *see also* aboriginal communities; native people
Indonesia 191
informal information 32, 47, 57–8, 67–8, 73, 144, 163, 191
informants 2, 16, 18, 64, 67, 69, 113, 148
informed consent *see* consent

insider knowledge 56, 58, 61–2, 65–6, 80
Institute of Development Studies 82
institutional prerogative 85, 88–9, 185
Institutional Review Boards (IRBs) 19,
    22, 113–14, 137–8, 153, 155–80; *see also*
    Ethical Review Panels, Research Ethics
    Boards/Committees
instrumental value 133
integrity of research 12, 22, 24, 57–8, 60–1,
    72, 76, 145, 166
intellectual disabilities 24–5, 58, 69–73,
    104–6, 122–6, 169
inter-subjectivities 86
internalisation 107
International Collaboration for
    Participatory Health Research (ICPHR)
    1–2, 4
International Monetary Fund (IMF) 81
International Participatory Research
    Network 3
internet 117, 169
intersectionality 24, 59, 76, 81, 85, 87, 94,
    201–3
interventions 1, 19, 63, 70, 73–5, 157, 165,
    194–5, 197
interviews 17–18, 36, 41, 47, 49–52; and
    blurred boundaries 59, 61, 67–72; and
    co-ownership 113, 117, 119–21, 123; and
    confidentiality 131, 139, 141–2, 145; and
    democratic representation 90, 92, 95–7;
    and review processes 159, 163–6, 169,
    172, 174–5; and social change 191, 195,
    198
intra-group conflict 5, 80–3, 85, 87, 94, 111
Inuit 4, 6, 24, 81, 95–7, 116
Iraq 191
Irish College of General Practitioners
    Research Ethics Committee 165
Irish Republic 19, 24–5, 58, 62, 73–6,
    165–7, 170–3
Islam 88
isolation 6, 18, 88, 146, 189, 191, 193–4,
    196, 204

jargon 109, 161, 166
Jervis, J. 155, 168–70

Kal, D. 103–4, 115, 119, 122, 125
Kalsem, K. 16, 25, 131–54
Kant, I. 10–12
Kaufman, C. 148
Kendall, C. 130
Kiijig Collective 117
kinship 84

Kothari, U. 59
Kral, M.J. 6, 80, 95–7
Kuriloff, P.J. 35
Kwartiermaken approach 104

Lalonde, C. 130
language issues 15–16, 21, 23, 64–5, 89;
    and co-ownership 108–9, 123–5; and
    confidentiality 133, 140; and review
    processes 161, 165–6; and social change
    192–3, 199
Latin America 90
leaders/leadership 33, 35, 37, 62, 80; and
    co-ownership 108, 113–14, 116–18, 120,
    126; and democratic representation 88–9,
    92–6, 99; and review processes 159, 161,
    163, 166–7; and social change 189, 192,
    196–7, 200–2
Ledwith, M. 184
legal researchers 132, 164, 174
legislation 7, 184, 189, 198–9, 204
life-worlds 34–7
Lincoln, Y. 34
literacy 3, 125, 140, 162
lived experience 59, 70–1, 104, 106,
    111; and co-ownership 116, 120; and
    confidentiality 139–40, 150; and review
    processes 176; and social change 181, 188,
    201, 203
lobbying 56
logistics 145, 194
logotherapy 74–6
London School of Economics 46–7
Lundy, P. 85–6

MacFarlane, A. 18, 24, 56–79, 155, 165–7
McGovern, M. 85-6
Mad Studies 105
Maguire, P. 4, 188
majoritarianism 84
managerialism 83, 106
managers 41–3
Mannell, J. 17, 31, 46–8
marginalisation 5, 24, 80, 88, 93; and co-
    ownership 104–5, 107, 111, 116, 119;
    and confidentiality 135, 138–9, 146; and
    review processes 174; and social change
    181, 188, 197–8
Marshall, Z. 130
Martin, A. 130
Marx, K. 83–4
Marxism 182
Matthies, A.-L. 103, 119–22
Mbatha, P. 181, 196–200

meaning-making 38, 73–4, 108–10
media 97, 109, 118, 120–1, 151, 164
mediation 6, 83, 140, 166
Medicines for Children Research Network (MCRN) 168
mental health 25, 43, 58, 105, 139–40, 173–6
Merritt, M. 135
Mertens, D. 191
Métis 116
Mexico 90
migrants 25, 89–92, 165–7, 181, 185, 193, 200–3
MIND 175
mind-mapping 67
Misereor 82
modernisation 97
Morocco 190
Multicultural Centre for Women's Health (MCWH) 200
multiculturalism 85, 182, 190–3, 200
Multiple Sclerosis (MS) 32
Muslims 87–8

narrative ethics 11–13
National Health Service (NHS) 168, 174–5
National Institute of Medical Research 113
National Institute of Mental Health 174
National Intercultural Health Strategy 62
Native Women's Association of Canada 117; see also Aboriginal communities, Indigenous people
Nazis 7, 13, 156
Netherlands 6, 18, 25, 32, 58, 69–73, 104, 122–5, 182, 189–93, 204
Netherlands Institute for Health Services Research (NIVEL) 70
Netherlands Organisation for Health Research and Development (ZonMw) 70
New Zealand 4
non-governmental organisations (NGOs) 19, 57, 82, 113–15, 120, 181, 194
norms/normativity 11, 13, 19, 82–3, 104, 112, 125, 176, 185
North, global 4, 11, 15–16, 82
North America 3–4
Nuremberg Code 7, 156
nurses/nursing 19, 24, 40–3, 58, 73, 75–6, 112, 168, 171–2
Nussbaum, M.C. 126

off-the-record information 58, 61, 69–73
Oliver, M. 44, 107

ontology 40, 182
oppression 1, 12, 21, 24, 91, 107, 119, 121, 162, 182, 184, 188, 204
outcomes 10, 14, 21, 25, 34–5; and blurred boundaries 56, 58; and co-ownership 110–12; and confidentiality 137, 146, 148, 153; and democratic representation 81, 86–7, 94–5; and power 37, 39, 49, 51; and review processes 171; and social change 182–3, 185–7, 190, 193, 199, 202, 204
outsiders 33, 37, 61, 80, 92, 105–6, 175, 199
ownership 9, 87, 103–30, 147, 149, 164

Pacific 181
palliative care 25, 170–1
paraplegia 32
Parent, W.A. 133
parents 25, 50–1, 86, 105, 121, 132, 147, 150–2, 156, 162, 168–70, 194
Participatory Action Groups (PAGs) 194–5
Participatory action research (PAR) 3, 80–86, 98, 119, 135, 152, 168; projects 25, 35
participatory health research (PHR) 4, 60, 146–9, 165–7
participatory learning and action (PLA) 4
Participatory Research for Health and Social Well-being 2
participatory research (PR) 3–5, 16–18, 59–62, 76–7, 103; and anonymity 131–54; approval of 165–7; and case collection 15–16; and co-ownership 103–30; and co-production 56–9; and community rights 80–102; and community role 5–7; and confidentiality 131–54; and conflict 80–102; degrees of participation 16–17; and democratic representation 80–102; and dissemination 103–30; emergent nature of 18–19; ethics in 1–30; and everyday ethics 20; and impact 103–30; and insider knowledge 66; and intellectual disabilities 69–73; participant burden 25, 100, 166, 170–3, 187–8; participant observations 58, 67, 69, 123; participation ladder 104–5; participatory mapping 17; participatory reflection and action 4; participatory rural appraisal 4; participatory theatre 24; participatory turn 3; participatory worldview 182, 188, 203; and patient experts 32; and points of action 63; and practice framework 20–2; and privacy 131–54; and review processes 155–80; and social change 181–203; and strengths of research 57

partnership 2–3, 5–6, 8–10, 15, 19–20; and blurred boundaries 57, 59–61, 68–9, 72, 76–7; and co-ownership 103, 106–10, 114–15; and confidentiality 139–40, 147–8, 152; and democratic representation 81, 90, 96–7; and ethics 24; and expectations 22, 32, 36–7; and power 31–55; and review processes 158–9, 161, 164, 167, 169; and social change 185, 188–9, 200–1

paternalism 135, 152, 173, 176

peasants 3

pedagogy 81, 87, 89, 100–1

peer researchers 9, 25, 59, 61–2, 65–6, 68–9, 139–42, 159

Peterman, M. 31–2, 42, 45, 48, 51

Philippines 25, 182, 186, 190, 194–6, 204

philosophy 10–13, 166, 171, 188

PhotoVoice 17, 19, 24, 58, 63, 73–6, 130, 138, 144–6, 150–2

phronesis 13

Plant, R. 5

pluralism 84

police 86, 95, 140–1

policy-makers 31, 34, 57–8, 77, 101; and co-ownership 107, 111–12, 115, 119–22; and social change 184, 189, 192–3, 198–9, 204

political science 116

politicians 58, 120–1

polity 84

pollution 116

Porter, S. 175

positionality 24, 67, 81, 85–7, 92, 97, 149, 181

positivism 35, 37–8, 155, 157, 176, 182

post-colonialism 182

poverty 5, 95, 139, 146, 195, 197

power 1, 6, 8, 13, 31–55; and co-ownership 103, 105–7, 125–6; and confidentiality 135, 137, 149; and democratic representation 80–1, 84, 87, 91, 93, 95–6; in Denmark 40–3; and ethics 21–2, 24–5; institutional power 185–6; power relations 31, 34, 42, 97, 134, 137–8, 189, 202–3; and review processes 169, 175; in Rwanda 44–9; and social change 181–2, 184–7, 189–90, 193, 199, 202–4; in UK 43–4, 49–52

Prainsack, B. 188

praxis 42, 86, 88, 182, 184, 203–4

precarity 48–9

priorities 32, 57, 98, 104, 108–11, 114, 118, 126, 186, 197

Pritchard, I. 136

privacy 2, 9–10, 25, 69, 111, 131–54, 158, 174, 176

privilege 24, 34, 38, 48, 80–1; and co-ownership 105, 107, 117, 119; and democratic representation 84, 93, 95; and social change 181, 186

protocols 36, 58, 64–6, 94, 113–16, 156–7, 160, 167, 173

proximity 11, 61–2

pseudonyms 132, 147–52

psychiatry 104–5

psychology 57, 181, 188

psychotherapy 74

PXE International 105

Qallunaat 24

Queensland University 150

race 34, 81, 85, 96, 160

radio stations 58, 66–8, 96

Ramarao, S. 148

reciprocity 40, 95, 109, 117, 189

recognition 146–9

recruitment 25, 44, 47, 49, 57–8; and blurred boundaries 62, 70, 73; and co-ownership 117; and confidentiality 139, 143–4; and democratic representation 90, 93; and review processes 159, 161–2, 166–7; and social change 194

reflection/reflexivity 4, 25, 35–6, 42, 46–7, 52; and blurred boundaries 58–9, 63, 66, 75–7; and co-ownership 107, 117, 123–4; and confidentiality 139, 142, 145, 149, 152; and democratic representation 86–7; and power 52; and review processes 164–7; and social change 181–2, 187–90, 193, 196, 199, 202–4

refugees 62, 181, 185, 200–3

relationality 1, 11, 13, 16, 20; and blurred boundaries 57, 59–60, 66, 68–9, 71–3, 76–7; and co-ownership 109, 111–12, 116–17, 119, 126; and confidentiality 133, 140, 143, 149; and democratic representation 82, 99; and power 46; power relations 31, 34, 42, 97, 134, 137–8, 189, 202–3; and review processes 155, 158; and social change 185–8, 191

religion 5, 11, 14, 85, 88–9, 191, 201

representation 5, 9, 20–1, 24, 80–102, 104–5, 108–9, 126

research assistants 17, 47, 116, 139, 200

research design 1, 6, 21, 50, 58; and blurred boundaries 67, 69, 71–2; and co-

ownership co-ownership 105, 117; and
confidentiality 134, 136, 139, 142–4, 147,
152; and democratic representation 81–2,
92–3; responsive research 123; and review
processes 159–60, 165–6, 168, 172,
175–6; and social change 183, 201, 203
Research and Development (R&D) 169
Research Ethics Boards (REB) 140, 142,
176; *see also* Institutional Review Boards;
Ethical Review Panels; Research Ethics
Committees
Research Ethics Committees (REC) 19,
22, 25, 135, 140, 142, 147, 165–8, 170–1,
174–6; *see also* Institutional Review
Boards; Ethical Review Panels; Research
Ethics Boards
Research Initiatives Bangladesh (RIB) 80,
86, 88
research proposals 23, 35–6, 48, 75–6, 117,
157, 161–2, 165–6, 168, 171–3
research teams 33, 62, 96, 109–10, 130; and
confidentiality 135–6, 138, 140–6; and
review processes 155, 158–62, 164, 173;
and social change 191, 201–2
resilience 49, 74, 141, 151, 167
resistance 43, 184, 188, 199
responsibility 7, 10–16, 20–1, 32–3, 35;
and blurred boundaries 62, 77; and co
-ownership 108, 113, 117, 121, 126; and
confidentiality 140, 142, 146, 149; and
power 39, 44–6, 49, 51–2; and social
change 184–5, 187, 189–93, 195–6,
201–2, 204
RESTORE project 165–7
review processes 1, 8–9, 19, 22, 155–80;
and blurred boundaries 75–7; and co-
ownership 113–15; and confidentiality
135, 137–8, 149, 153; and ethics 25; and
power 35
Richman, K.A. 61
rigour 57, 59, 61, 66
ripple effects 57, 59, 72, 76, 110
risks 8, 22, 32, 37–9, 42; and blurred
boundaries 62; and co-ownership 106,
111, 119, 122, 126; and confidentiality
132, 136, 138, 141–2, 148–51; and
democratic representation 93; and power
48, 50–1; and review processes 156–8,
160–5, 167, 169–70, 172, 176; and social
change 183, 187, 189–90, 192
Robinson, J. 31, 38, 43–6
Roche, B. 18, 24, 56–79
roles 1, 6, 9, 13, 18; and blurred boundaries
56, 58–63, 71–2, 75–7; and co-ownership

117; and confidentiality 143–4; and
democratic representation 93; and power
33–4, 36, 50; and review processes 158–9,
176; and social change 186, 201
Roma people 6, 24, 96–100
Routledge, P. 184
Russo, J. 106–7
Rwanda 17, 24, 32, 191

Satchwell, C. 17, 31, 49–51
scandals 7
schizophrenia 106
segregation 82, 174
service users 25, 31, 42, 46, 77, 104–9,
119–23, 141, 158, 173–6
sex workers 90–1, 106, 156
sexuality 5, 21, 34
Shabangu, P. 16, 56, 64–6
shakti-shamavay 87
shared vision 39, 42
Shore, N. 35
Sightsavers International (SSI) 113
silence 81, 85–6, 89–92, 105
slow movement 40, 52
social capital 58, 66
social change/social action 10, 21, 25,
57, 181–203; and blurred boundaries
62–3; and co-ownership 103, 110, 112,
121–2; conceptualisation of 183–5; and
confidentiality 134, 138, 151–2; and
power 39–40, 42, 48, 185–7; and review
processes 159
social contract 84
social exclusion 122, 175; Social Exclusion
Unit 174 *see also* exclusion
social justice 1, 3–4, 25, 34, 37; and co-
ownership 106, 110, 116–17, 126; and
democratic representation 83, 87, 93, 95;
and review processes 156, 163; and social
change 182–3, 186, 188, 200–3
social media 69, 117, 121
Social Model of Disability 44
social movements 3, 151, 184, 196, 200
social relations 24, 36, 57, 61–4, 77, 184
social sciences 8, 57, 87, 156
social workers 143, 155, 181
socialism 86
sociology 3, 57
solidarity 5, 11–12, 25, 119, 182, 187–90,
193, 196, 199–200, 202–4
Soo Chan Carusone 131, 143
South, global 11, 15–16, 82
South Africa 25, 182, 186, 190, 196–200,
204

Southern Africa 16, 24–5, 58, 64–6
Spanish language 90–1
stakeholders 4, 17, 33, 39, 51; and blurred
  boundaries 56–7, 60; and co-ownership
  104, 106, 108–10, 112–13; and
  confidentiality 133–4, 153; and review
  processes 156, 165–6, 168–9, 175–6; and
  social change 182, 188
status 21, 24, 34, 38, 60; and blurred
  boundaries 62, 65–6; and confidentiality
  140–1, 144; and democratic
  representation 84, 89, 93, 100; and review
  processes 172; and social change 185,
  199
stereotypes 38, 117
stewardship 37, 164
stigmatisation 5, 34, 37, 81, 88; and co-
  ownership 108–9, 111, 122, 126; and
  confidentiality 139, 141; and democratic
  representation 98; and review processes
  161, 164, 175
stories 11–19, 37–38, 61, 68, 73–75, 111,
  172, 192; Stories to Connect 49; see also
  narrative ethics
Strike, C. 130, 143
structural inequalities/injustice 35, 84, 87,
  97, 103; and co-ownership 110, 121; and
  social change 181–4, 189, 191–3, 196,
  200, 204
Sub-Saharan Africa 15
subalterns 83
substance use 139, 143–4, 156
suicide 9, 81, 95–7
supervisors 81, 92–3, 101, 147, 190–1
Sussex University 82
sustainability 21–2, 25, 32–3, 39, 113,
  117–18, 182, 184–5, 189, 196, 199, 204
Swantz, M.-L. 3
Swaziland 25, 130, 146–9
Switzer, S. 130, 143
synergies 75–6

Tandon, R. 3
Tanzania 3, 25, 104, 112–15
technocracy 81
tensions 5, 9, 16, 24, 34; and blurred
  boundaries 57, 59–62, 75, 77; and
  co-ownership 112, 120, 124; and
  confidentiality 131, 136, 138, 146–9; and
  democratic representation 80–1, 88–9,
  93–4, 97–101; and power 36, 49; and
  review processes 155, 157–8, 175–6; and
  social change 182, 191, 197, 204
Teunissen, T. 103–4, 115, 119, 122, 125

theatre 86; see also Boal's Theatre of the
  Oppressed
theology 188
therapeutic processes 19, 24, 59, 63, 73–6,
  143–5
timelines 8, 22, 32, 36–7, 162, 186
tokenism 52, 82
Toronto Teen Survey Team 156
Toronto University 116, 143
training 35, 44, 47, 49, 62; and blurred
  boundaries 64–5, 77; and co-ownership
  123; and confidentiality 136, 139, 153;
  and review processes 155, 159, 174; and
  social change 202
translation 15, 21, 62, 109, 124–5, 140,
  166
trust 8, 11, 22, 32, 34; and blurred
  boundaries 58, 67, 76; and co-ownership
  115; and confidentiality 131, 133–5,
  138, 141–2, 144–5, 152; and democratic
  representation 100; and power 37–9,
  41–2; and review processes 159, 161–2,
  166, 176; and social change 189, 198,
  201
truth-telling 85–6
Turkey 190–1
Turner, K. 107
Tuskegee Syphilis experiment 7, 13, 156
tutors 169

unemployed people 34, 48, 104, 119–21,
  194
UNESCO 197
unintended consequences 62, 68, 72, 75
Union for Public Employees 41
United Kingdom (UK) 4, 14, 18, 24–5, 32,
  46, 66, 81–2, 135, 168–70, 173–6
United States (US) 4, 7, 95, 112, 114–15,
  170
University of Central Lancashire 49
university researchers 33, 44, 58, 69–71, 81,
  97, 100, 111, 119, 122–5
Upshur, R. 157
utilitarianism 11–12

Van den Bosch, R. 103, 122–5
Van den Hoonaard, W.C. 8, 135
Van Zuijlen, R. 31–2, 42, 45, 48, 51
Vaughan, C. 10, 25, 181–203
vested interests 103
vice 202
Vietnam 25, 130, 150–2
violence 24–5, 46–9, 84–5, 106, 182, 185,
  195, 200–3

virtue *see* ethics, virtue
voice 1, 4, 17, 21, 24; and blurred
    boundaries 66; and co-ownership
    103–6, 117, 119–22; and confidentiality
    135, 137–8, 152; and democratic
    representation 82–3, 85–6, 92–4; and
    power 33, 39, 42; and review processes
    175; and social change 184–5, 189, 192,
    198, 200–2
Vu Song Ha 130, 150–2
VU University Medical Centre 32, 104
vulnerable people 25, 33, 35, 37–8, 46; and
    blurred boundaries 69; and co-ownership
    105; and confidentiality 152; and
    democratic representation 89–90; and
    power 49; and review processes 157, 160,
    166–7, 169–74; and social change
    191–3

Ward, L. 83
Welch, S.D. 119, 122, 126
well-being 1–2, 11, 14, 20, 31, 95–7, 174,
    183
West 32, 48
Western Europe 43

White people 32, 64, 92, 95–7, 104, 181,
    190
Wiebe, S.M. 18–19, 103, 116–19
Wilkinson, C. 17–18, 56, 66–8
Willowbrook State School 156
Wolf, L.E. 157
women 3, 5–6, 18–19, 25, 46–8; and blurred
    boundaries 64; and co-ownership
    113–14, 117; and confidentiality 135,
    137; and democratic representation 82–3,
    90–1, 93, 96; and review processes 160;
    and social change 181–2, 185–6, 189,
    191–6, 200–3
workshops 40–1, 64–5, 73, 147, 175
World Bank 81
World Heritage Sites 197
World War, Second, 7

York, K. 103, 112–15
Yoshihama, M. 186
young people 49–51, 96, 117–22, 132, 135,
    150–2, 156, 159–60, 162, 168–70
YouTube 118

Zambia 24, 80, 92–5